200 Tips Every Runner Should Know

Train Smarter, Reduce Injuries, and
Become a Better Runner

GRADY CASH

For information about special discounts, bulk purchases, or speaking engagements, contact the author at gradycash@gmail.com.

Copyright © 2018 Grady Cash
All rights reserved.
ISBN: 978-0-9998934-0-1
1. Heath 2. Exercise & Fitness 3. Running
Printed in the United States of America
Gerodemocracy Press

Praise for this Book

A well-written treasure trove of Running Tips! Extremely accessible and useful suggestions. This is a "Must Have," reference manual that can improve many facets of your running experience. Grady has done the legwork. Now, you can draw on his knowledge to improve your training and have a better understanding of the full spectrum of issues involved in the process.

- Roger Pierce, age 72, 11 Masters Track World Records, 18 USA Records from 60m to 400m, 15 Gold Medals at World Championships, 38 Golds at USA Masters Championships over the past 33 years. Inducted into the USATF Masters Hall of Fame in 2008. Still actively competing as an elite Masters Sprinter and Coach.

This book is like a cheat code to the runner's craft! The insights that Grady Cash offers here have been tested in the only laboratory that counts -- out on the roads, in training, and in competition. Written in a friendly and accessible style, never didactic and always encouraging, this book seems to have the answer to every problem that a runner may encounter. This is a national class book from a national class runner. Mr. Cash has accomplished something quite tremendous, distilling 40 years of practical experience and deep thinking into a simple and clear guide for all runners.

- Jeff Edmonds, 2:35 marathoner. 3:59 1500m. 15:04 5K. 1st overall, Avenue of the Giants and Flying Monkey marathons. Coach for many years, including a high school state champion team and coaching countless individuals to personal bests. Blogs on running at LogicOfLongDistance.com.

Grady displays an encyclopedic knowledge of running and do-it-yourself ingenuity. The mix makes for an informative and fun read.

- Margie Stoll, gold medalist, National Senior Games. World ranked, F70 1500 meters.

Grady's prudent approach to the management of injuries is one that evades even the most talented and seasoned athletes. These tips offer terrific insight on staying healthy, understanding your own body, and maximizing the enjoyment of our sport.

- Jeannette Faber, 21st, 2012 Olympic Trials Marathon, 2:36.50. Several marathon gold medals, including 2012 Twin Cities Marathon in 2:32:37. Bronze, 2011 USA 25K Championships. Cross Country All American.

I wish this book had been available when I started running 38 years ago. I've run as a heel striker all this time. After reading Grady's marvelous book, I am transitioning to a forefoot strike, which has already improved my racing. This is only one of many tips which I found extremely helpful in this well-written book. Thank you, Grady, for sharing your wisdom and training expertise to help runners who want to excel and run the best they can.

- Carlos Cobos, age 78. Runner for 38 years. 2015 National Senior Games: Silver in 800m, Bronze in 10K. 2012 Boston Marathon finisher. Tennessee individual age and age group records: 800m, 1500m, 1 mile, 4 miles, & 8 miles. 1st in age group at 2016 Rock 'n Roll Nashville Half Marathon, 2nd in age group at 2014 Peachtree 10K.

Grady Cash is a legend in our running groups. If you have a question or problem, "Just ask Grady." I had the pleasure of meeting Grady at the Senior Olympics. At age 58, I was new to running and open to advice from "the experts." We became training partners, and over the last five years, I have had the distinct advantage of his wisdom, which you are about to discover in this book. Without his mentoring, encouragement, insight, and friendship, I could not have obtained the level of success I have reached in my short running career.

- David Schmanski, M60 World Record 4x800m, American Record 400m, 2015 Ranked #1 in the World—200m, 400m, and 800m. 11-time National Champion, 27-time USATF Masters All American.

After 50 years of running and some years of team and personal coaching, I am learning things from Grady as a coach I never knew. I am very impressed by the scope of his new and wonderful book. This book is so unique and helpful that it should be on the shelf of every runner in the country. It is not only a great reference book, but it's also just fun, enlightening reading.

- Ted Wilson, age 80, 50 years running experience, 3 Boston marathons, 3 Half Ironman Triathlons. Ran 1500m in 4:36 at age 51, TN M80 champion in 200, 400, 800 and 1500m. M80 state record, 800m.

Grady Cash knows what he is talking about! An experienced runner, a champion competitor, and a humble sportsman, Grady is always willing to share his experience and help anyone get the most of their training and running. Pick up this book, lace up your shoes, and take your best run!

- Bob VanFleteren, 2015 Nat'l Sr Games, 50M, 100M, Long Jump, High Jump

After 30+ years of running, I thought I had learned every tip and strategy. Not only did I gain several new ideas from this book, but I was also reminded of ways to make running fun again.

- Diane Vilimek, runner, triathlete and middle school running coach

Very thoughtful and well written. It's obvious that Grady dedicated significant time and energy to put this project together over many years. The outcome is a book with great depth and a wealth of information incredibly useful to any runner. A great gift to the running community.

- Sue McCarthy, 15 USA Masters gold medals, American record USA Masters Track and Field Club 4x400 Relay, National Senior Games Record 50m, 5 Corporate Track and Field Records, 3 Maine Senior Games Records, 3rd in the world 2015 100m (1st in the US)

What an enjoyable read! I would recommend this book to any runner, regardless of experience—from weekend-warrior to grizzled track vet. Grady has accumulated a vast wealth of knowledge over countless miles logged on the road, track, and trails. He graciously shares this knowledge with his readers with interesting stories and humorous anecdotes. In addition to more than 200 running tips, there are thought-provoking sections on biomechanics and nutrition. Beyond the standard "how to dress for cold weather running," Grady includes tips on how to make your own orthotics and where to find inexpensive prescription sunglasses. This is valuable advice you won't find in your average running book. In a genre sorely lacking in originality, Grady has added something new and truly worth reading.

Ted Towse, Ph.D. Pres, Nashville Harriers. 5k PR: 14:58.

Grady's book is an amazing reference for all runners from young to old, whether beginner or veteran, social to competitive. His passion for our sport flows out of every topic he addresses and his expertise from years of experience and research is sound advice. I found several tips to be things I learned the hard way. Now runners have all they need at their fingertips in this book!

-   Diana Bibeau, 118 marathons (5 Boston). 25 years running in road races from 5K to marathon. Past President, Nashville Striders Running Club

Grady Cash is a valuable asset to any running community. Not only does he bring an encouraging, uplifting, and contagious positive attitude to any running group, he also has a wealth of knowledge and the kindness and willingness to support his fellow runners. In 200 Tips Every Runner Should Know, Grady shares his secrets to success with the running community at large in an easily digestible, enjoyable format. I would recommend this book to any runner striving to achieve their goals.

-   Joseph Elsakr, Former Division 1 athlete, Duke University. 2:23:32 marathon PR. Other PRs: 1:07:42 half marathon; 31:17, 10k; 15:11, 5k; and 4:33, mile.

Here is what Nashville runners know: If you have a question about any aspect of running, no matter how arcane or how technical, whether about training pace, running injury, or cold weather, Grady Cash has the answer, or at least an informed opinion. He is a student of the sport. He has not just read it and remembered it and re-read it, he has lived it, lived it in countless training runs ground out along trails through the woods and around university tracks, lived it through countless road races, and track meets dotting numerous states. From that base of knowledge and experience, he has distilled like Tennessee sipping whiskey this informative gem of a book.

- Dallas Smith, author, *Falling Forward*, M65 TN state records in 5k, 4mi, 8k, 10k, 15k, 10mi, 13.1mi, and marathon

A great handbook for beginners and veterans alike. I especially like the chapter with tips about buying running shoes. I wish this chapter could be handed to every new customer that walks through the door of a specialty running store looking for proper footwear. As a competitive runner since I was 14, it's easy from time to time to get caught in a rut. Grady's contagious search for improvement and joy within the sport has always been a constant reminder that the sport of running isn't a task or a job to get through each day, but a rewarding part of life that shouldn't be taken for granted.

- Hunter Hall, Marketing Director, Fleet Feet Nashville, (2014, 2015, 2016 Top 50 Running Store in the Country, Competitor *Magazine*). 2:33 Marathoner (Indianapolis Monumental 2015). 1st Place- Chattanooga Mountains Stage Race 2016

Table of Contents

Acknowledgements

Running is more fun in a group, and my friends have helped make writing this book more fun as well. I'd like to thank those who contributed ideas to make this a better book: Marshall Albritton, Karen Austin, Diana Bibeau, Bob Buckholz, Brad Bradshaw, Janna Dedman, Mike DeMerritt, Sean Donahue, Nick Ged, Sue Anne Perry, Bill Menees, Kelly Murphy, Frank Possinger, John Spencer, Trent Rosenbloom, Tony Recker, Christi Seckman, Dallas Smith, Margie Stoll, Paul Scalisi, Charlie Taylor, Diane Vilimek, Ted Wilson, and Phil Zimmerman

And a very special thanks to those who have helped me on my journey to become a better runner. Peter Pressman, President of the Nashville Striders for providing such a great environment for Nashville runners. Jim Spivey, 3-time Olympian, who gave me the confidence to compete at the national level. The late Randy Sturgeon, former owner of National Masters News, for encouraging me to run masters track. The great staff at the Tennessee Senior Olympics who made it a joy to participate and make new friends each year. Personal trainers Rick Munoz, Daniel Johnson, and Patrick Sullivan who taught me proper lifting technique. Vanderbilt personal trainer Johnny Pryor and his noon running group. World champion Roger Pierce for sharing his workouts and literally giving me the shirt off his back for our 4x400m world record relay. My fellow relay members who helped me set a new world record: Charles Allie, Roger Pierce, and Noah Perlis. And a very special thanks to training partners who gave me the motivation to run on dreary days and encouragement to write this book: John Thorpe, Sherri Hahn, Susan Lambreth, and fellow world record holder David Schmanski.

Introduction

As a runner for over 40 years, I've been around the block a few times—make that a few thousand times—and along the way, I learned a lot about running.

Many of these lessons were learned by painful trial and error because information on them simply didn't exist. Fortunately, you won't have to make those mistakes. You can learn from my experience, but that's not the only reason why I wrote this book.

In 1998, I suffered a severe running injury. Several doctors, including two at the Mayo Clinic, told me that I could never run again. There was nothing they could do. My running days were over.

It was horrific news—the sport that I had loved and taken for granted was gone. My need for an adrenalin boost spiraled out of control. Over the next two years, I bought three motorcycles and a supercharged sports car, but they couldn't fill the void left by the loss of my beloved sport.

By 2000, I'd had enough of life without running. Against doctors' advice, I laced up my shoes and headed out the door. It hurt—sometimes it hurt a lot. I'd have to walk until the pain went away, but when it did, I'd start up again at a turtle's pace. In two months, I could run three miles without stopping. In three months, the pain was gone. I was a runner again! It wasn't heroic on my part. It was just that the pain of not running was worse than the temporary discomfort I felt when running.

Probably the injury had healed over time, leaving behind scar tissue. When I returned to running, the scar tissue stretched a little with each step. Finally, I was able to run—really run—for the first time in years.

It was a great personal victory—I had won back my favorite pastime, and I would never take it for granted again. I became a runner once more, but the time I lost could never be recaptured.

At age 53, training harder wasn't the solution, so I immersed myself in everything I could read about our sport. I became a student in the art of running. *I resolved to train smarter.* I read everything I could find on running. I taught myself how to convert from heel to forefoot strike years before it became a hot topic. I invented and filed a patent on a new type of running gear. I created a way for runners to make their own orthotics.

But thanks to my career-threatening injury and recovery, I never lost sight of the essence of the sport—the sheer joy of running. That is the secret to becoming a lifelong runner. *Running has to be fun.* If you avoid the mistakes described in this book, running can grant you lifetime benefits that multiply as you get older. Many of my running friends in their 50s are strikingly youthful when compared to their peers—and remarkably healthy.

The typical 65-year-old is on three prescription drugs and has at least one chronic illness. At age 70, I'm still healthy. Investing in running is like buying health insurance at a discount.

There's no reason beginners reading this book can't be like me. Just make it a priority in your life. This book is here to help you. Just one of the tips might change your running career, so let's get started, beginning with the secrets of the perfect shoe.

1

Becoming a Better Runner

When I first started running, I wasn't very good. I failed to make my high school track team. I didn't run in college. When I started running local races in my thirties, I would typically finish outside the top three in my age group. In short, I was like most of the readers of this book. Yet as I write this, I've become one of the fastest masters runners in the world, setting a new world record in the 4x400m relay in 2018.

What happened that allowed me to find this remarkable success? I certainly didn't get an infusion of talent in my old age. My genetics didn't change. Sure, I was training hard, but so was my competition. How did I improve so much?

The catalyst for my improvement occurred twenty years ago when two doctors at the Mayo Clinic told me I could never run again. It took me two years to heal enough to resume running, but when I did, I resolved to never take my favorite sport for granted. I became a student in the art of running, reading everything I could find and joining a running club with a 3-time Olympian as my coach. I couldn't change my genetics, nor could I turn back the clock, but I could still optimize every aspect of my training to become the best runner I could be.

Here's the good news. You won't have to hire an Olympian or run tens of thousands of miles to learn these lessons. They've been carefully organized by category for you. If you're injured, you can just flip to the chapter on injuries to find the best way to rehab. If you're buying new shoes, Chapter 2 will show you common mistakes to avoid.

More than 200 tips in this book!

By the way, the title is just a catchy hook to get runners to pick up the book. *200 Tips Every Runner Should Know* contains more than 200 numbered tips and over 40 bonus tips. Plus, some tips have as many as a half dozen separate tips within that tip's topic. Based on counting a random sample of tips, you'll find over 400 individual running hacks in this book, so don't get hung up on the number.

Granted, if you've been running a while, you'll already know some of these tips, but what if you learn something that saves you several weeks of rehab? What if the speed tips shave a few minutes off your next marathon so you can qualify for Boston? Those tips alone could justify your investment in buying this book.

Beginners often wonder why they get injured, why they can't lose weight, why they can't run faster, or why they can't stay motivated to run. Well, it's not your fault.

Thousands of runners are like King Sisyphus from Greek mythology—forced to push a boulder to the top of the mountain only to have it roll down before they reach the peak. These modern-day versions of Sisyphus are frustrated by constant injuries or the inability to get faster in spite of hard training. As a result, they never become the runners they could be.

The problem is that running is supposedly so easy that anyone can do it with no training. You just put one foot in front of the other, right?

Thus, beginners don't get much training in actually running. They just start with whatever shoes they have and little to no guidance on running form.

As a result, *learning how to run is typically a reactive process.* You run, you do something wrong, and if you're lucky, your body adapts to it. If not, you just continue to make those same mistakes, never getting faster, never losing weight, and constantly getting injured.

Compare this to other sports—tennis or golf, for example. Beginners don't go on a tennis court until they have lessons. Golfers often spend hours perfecting their swing, but running is different.

Beginners are told to get a good pair of shoes (without really knowing what that means) and then go for a group run with 20 other similarly clueless individuals in various stages of learning the sport. If you're part of an informal training group, other than receiving a training schedule, there's very little guidance on how to actually run.

If you are injured or not getting faster, it's not your fault. No one taught you how to run.

If you survive past this level, the sport is still reactive. Even if you hire a coach, you won't get advice on injuries until *after* you get injured. There's very little proactive advice to prevent injuries from occurring in the first place.

Over half of runners training for their first half or full marathon drop out due to injuries. It's no wonder so many people leave the sport! No one is teaching them how to become a better runner. Instead, they're forced to learn through the painful process of trial and error, only learning how to prevent a common running injury *after* it occurs.

Not surprisingly, they eventually get injured, or their body adapts to poor shoes and poor running form, which in turn prevents them from getting faster.

The good news is that you can avoid these injuries and mistakes. In this book, you'll learn my favorite tips distilled from over 40 years of running to help you avoid injuries, recover from injuries faster, improve your running form, race faster, and stay more comfortable while running.

After all, if you're freezing on your next winter run or losing training time due to a nagging little injury, you're not happy, and you're not becoming a better runner.

Unconventional Format: Conventional style spells out single digit numbers as words, but runners typically use numerals when referring to reps, sets, paces, and distances even when the number is a single digit. This book uses numerals for single digit times, paces, distances, reps, sets, and weights. Other single digit numbers will be spelled out.

What's Not in This Book: If you're looking for training plans—Couch to 5K or 18-week Marathon Training—there are other excellent books for that purpose. They'll be listed in Recommended Readings at the end of this book.) Instead, this book focuses on tips you need to know to make your training successful, regardless of the training plan you choose or your current fitness.

After all, a training plan only provides daily workouts. It doesn't tell you what you should be doing before, during, and after those workouts to get the most out of your training time.

Finally, I am like you. I'm not an Olympian to whom running came easily. I'm a modestly talented runner who never ran in high school or college who became one of the fastest masters runners in the world by applying the secrets in this book—secrets you will soon learn.

Let's begin by learning the secrets of the perfect shoe.

2

Secrets of the Perfect Shoe

Shoes are your most important running gear, yet even veteran runners make mistakes in their choice of running shoes. In a one-hour training run, your shoes hit the ground over 10,000 times, transferring about three times your body weight with each foot strike to your feet, arches, shins, knees, and hips. If the shoe doesn't fit properly, each impact twists ligaments and tendons in ways they shouldn't be twisted. The result can be a myriad of running injuries.

The challenge is that feet are like snowflakes. No two are alike. Some runners have narrow feet; others have wide feet. Some runners have very high arches; some have normal arches, and some have flat feet. Shoe manufacturers attempt to address these problems by making different types of shoes—motion control, stability, cushion, neutral, performance, racing, and minimalist, and so on—but there are billions of uniquely shaped feet and only a few dozen shapes of running shoes.

Here's a secret that manufacturers don't publicize about running shoes.

1.   Running Shoes Aren't Made to Fit You

A few years back I had the opportunity to become co-owner of a running store. Ultimately that venture fell through, but as part of the startup process I met with most of the major shoe manufacturers and tested dozens of different shoes. I was initially surprised to discover that none of these shoes were perfect for me.

Here's a secret most runners don't know. *Running shoes are not made to fit you.* Instead, shoes are made to fit the most runners possible within their particular niche. From a business perspective, that makes sense. Manufacturers want their shoes to fit many runners as possible within that shoe's target market.

As a result, the arches of almost all running shoes are too low. If they were made to fit the average arched runner, the arch would be too high to fit 50% of their target market.

If your arch is strong enough, poor arch support may not be a problem, but as you increase mileage, poor arch support can cause injuries. Common arch-related injuries include plantar fasciitis, Achilles tendinitis, runners knee, shin splints, IT band syndrome, and more.

The arches of most running shoes are too low.

Shoe manufacturers compensate for this by creating beefy motion control and stability shoes, but these shoes have their own set of problems. They're heavy, inflexible, unresponsive, and mask problems with poor running form.

A better solution is to correct any form flaws and wear a lighter, neutral shoe, adding just enough extra arch support for your unique foot. You'll learn how to improve your form and add arch support to shoes in an upcoming chapter.

Granted, an off-the-shelf shoe can sometimes come pretty close to perfect, just as an off-the-rack suit can provide a reasonably good fit, but chances are the shoes you like best are going to have some little nagging flaw. The toe box is too tight. It causes a blister on your arch. You pronate too much. The list is endless. Most runners can vouch for this because they've found shoes they thought were perfect, only to find out their shoes caused a problem after running in them for a few days.

Since feet are like snowflakes, you aren't going to find a shoe that's custom-made to fit you. With that in mind, you can avoid shoe-related injuries and get a shoe that works for your unique foot and running form by following the steps in this chapter.

2.   Think of Shoe Expenses as Insurance

Some runners think nothing of spending $1,000 for room, hotel, and registration to run a marathon, but then they balk at spending $150 to replace shoes that might be causing an injury.

Honestly, I used to feel the same way until I had a serious running injury a few years ago. It wasn't responding to conventional treatments. It would get better for a while and then I'd have a relapse. I spent nearly $1,000 to go to the 2013 USATF Indoor Masters Championships, but I couldn't even warm up properly and finished second in the 800 meters. I limped home and spent several weeks in physical therapy. Worse, I was left to wonder if the outcome would have been different if I had gone to the starting line uninjured.

Finally, I had an epiphany. Rather than continue to spend weeks in physical therapy and incur related out-of-pocket expenses, I decided to see if changing shoes could make a difference. Instead of testing just one shoe, I resolved to test every running shoe I could get my hands on to see if new shoes could fix the injury.

It worked. I didn't even have to test that many shoes. I just started by assuming something similar to what I was already wearing wouldn't help so I would need to go to something radically different. To be fair, it didn't resolve the problem immediately, but I was able to resume training. Over time the injury went away thanks to a radical change in shoes.

This isn't an unusual occurrence. I talked with a world record holder in my age group who not only had a similar experience; he was wearing the same shoe!

Another friend, also a world record holder, had a similar heel problem. I suggested he could resolve it by switching to the Hoka Bondi, a newer version of the shoe I was wearing. The unique rocker sole of these shoes deserves your consideration if you have chronic injuries. They're discussed in more detail in Chapter 5 "Preventing Common Running Injuries."

My point is that instead of spending weeks going to a physical therapist, see if a change of shoes or orthotics might help.

By the way, I'm not knocking physical therapists. They can be great, as can chiropractors, masseurs, and sports medicine professionals. What I am saying is that when injuries occur, rather than just treating the symptoms, look for the underlying cause of the problem. A good place to start is with your shoes.

Good shoes are like buying running insurance.

Running is one the least expensive of all sports. Golfers, for example, can easily spend $1,000 for clubs and even more for greens fees and memberships. Cyclists can expect to invest over $2,000 for a good road bike, shoes, and other gear. Running, by comparison, requires only a good pair of running shoes, so don't skimp on shoes. My current shoes retail for $150, but I much prefer that to the expense of medical treatments and the loss of training time. Oh, and you're going to learn how to buy your shoes much cheaper than that in Chapter 18 "Money Saving Tips."

3. The #1 Mistake in Buying Shoes

Most local running stores are staffed by veteran runners. Overwhelmingly, they will attest to the accuracy of this tip. Runners, even many experienced runners, tend to buy running shoes that are too small.

Running shoes can vary a full size from dress or casual shoes. This creates problems for runners who mistakenly think they should wear the same size running shoe as a regular shoe. This is especially true for women, who are accustomed to wearing very tight-fitting shoes without socks. For example, a woman who typically wears a size 9 goes to buy her first pair of running shoes, but she is shocked to discover that the size 9 fits very snug. Since she normally wears a size 9, she buys it anyway, often against the advice of the sales staff.

Unfortunately, this is not just a vanity issue. Shoes that are too small can cause a myriad of foot injuries, including Morton's Neuroma, black toenails, and blisters on the toes.

Shoes that are too small can cause injuries.

The lesson here is to buy shoes that fit, regardless of the claimed size. It sounds obvious, but it's amazing how many runners fail to follow this simple rule.

Running shoes should be bigger than casual shoes because feet can swell a half size during exercise and because the toes need more room to move around. Also, running socks that are thicker than your normal sock can add a half size to shoe fit.

"I used to wear a size 9 or sometimes a 9½ in a dress shoe," says Kelly M, a six-time All American in cross country and track. "Now, all my running shoes are 10½. I never worry about the size. No one can see the size anyway. Plus, some running shoes run a half size to a full size too small."

You think that I would be immune to this problem. Not so. A few years back I heard great things about a particular racing flat. I tried on a 9, but it was too small. I tried the 9½, but it was also too small. I tried a 10. It was close, but it was too narrow in the toe box, a common problem for me. Disappointed, I left to walk around the Expo, but before leaving, I decided to give the shoe one more test run. I went back and tried on a 10½—I've never worn a 10½ in any shoe in my life—and it fit. I bought the shoe and loved it.

Bonus Tip: With most running injuries, the first suspect is shoes. Are your shoes worn out? Even the best running shoes last only 300-500 miles. Keep a running log or journal and track the miles on your shoes so you can replace them before problems occur.

4. Buy Shoes at Running Stores

Stores that specialize in selling running shoes and apparel will usually have veteran runners on staff who can help find the right shoe for you. Plus, you can test drive your new shoes before buying them. Some running stores even have treadmills and offer runners a free gait analysis. *The money you might save by buying online is wasted if you get injured from a poorly fitted shoe.* Some running stores provide generous return privileges. Be sure to ask about this because sometimes fit problems only show up after you've worn the shoe a few times.

Bonus Tip: Don't assume the same shoe model will fit you next year. Manufacturers routinely change their shoes from one year to the next.

A veteran marathoner who had worn the same model of shoe for several years developed foot problems. "I went to a running store for a free gait analysis on a treadmill and learned the arch support was too low for my foot," said Sherri H, a veteran of the New York, Boston, Chicago, and Paris marathons. "I had been wearing the wrong shoe for years, and eventually it caught up to me. They recommended a different shoe and the problems disappeared almost immediately."

5.   A Common Mistake When Trying on Shoes

You'd think veteran runners should know this, but sales staff tell me runners often try on shoes without their normal running socks and orthotics. The wrong sock can make a big difference in whether a shoe fits properly. The difference between a very thin sock and a normal cushioned running sock can add a half-size to the shoes you wear.

Carry your normal running socks and orthotics (if you wear them) with you when trying on new shoes. This is especially important for women who often don't normally wear socks with their dress or casual shoes. By the way, if you wear orthotics, you'll learn how to save hundreds in an upcoming chapter by making your own. It's easy. I've made them for friends while still at the track after a workout.

---

*Don't forget your orthotics and running socks
when trying on running shoes.*

Bonus Tip: It's a good idea to take your old running shoes with you. An experienced salesperson can look at the wear pattern on your old shoes, diagnose imbalances, and recommend a shoe to avoid future injuries due to that imbalance.

Bonus Tip: When buying shoes, you should also consider off-the-shelf orthotics and different socks. It's a great time to try orthotics because you can test them in a brand-new shoe. If you always run in the same type of socks, you might be amazed at how much difference a different sock can make. You'll learn more about socks in Chapter 9 "Comfort." Be sure to read it before buying new shoes and socks.

The right socks can make a difference in shoe fit.

---

6. Secrets of Fitting the Wide Foot

If you have a wide foot, you can buy a EE shoe, but that greatly limits your shoe choices. Also, if you have a wide forefoot and narrow heel as I do, an EE width shoe will slip up and down in the heel. If your foot is wide mostly in the forefoot, you might solve the problem by buying shoes with a wider toe box. If that doesn't work, here are some additional tips.

First, wear extremely thin socks. If that doesn't make the shoe wide enough, replace the factory insert with a thinner insert. My favorite insert for this purpose is the Superfeet Black off-the-shelf orthotic. It's a very thin insert that also provides some arch support.

Another approach is to skip the bottom eyelets when lacing the shoe to allow it to stretch in the forefoot. There are more tips on how to make the forefoot of your shoes wider in Chapter 5 "Preventing Common Running Injuries."

Women Runners: If you have a wide foot, consider wearing a men's shoe. Many of the color combinations are gender-neutral. If the shoe slips on your heel, you can resolve that problem with butterfly lacing or elastic laces. Both types of lacing are explained in Chapter 5.

7. Secrets of Fitting the Narrow Foot

If you have a narrow foot, the advice is almost a mirror image of what you've just read for the wide foot. First, wear a thicker sock. Next, use a thicker shoe insert. The Superfeet Green is a relatively thick insert, and they make even thicker ones. You'd be surprised how much difference an extra millimeter of insert cushioning can make in shoe fit.

I've mentioned Superfeet twice now because of my firsthand experience with them, but other companies also make excellent off-the-shelf orthotics. Ask your running store salesperson for help in finding the right one for you. Finally, men with very narrow feet should consider women's running shoes. Many shoe models are available in gender-neutral colors. You'll need to size up about 1½ sizes.

8. Increase Shoe Life by 30%

As sports go, running is relatively inexpensive, but if you buy several pairs of shoes a year, the cost can add up. Here are five ways to increase the life of your shoes by up to 30% or more.

1. Rotate Shoes: By alternating shoes each day, the cushioning has more time to recover between runs. More important, alternating reduces the risk of shoe-related injuries. Since each model of shoe fits a little differently, rotating shoes gives the foot a rest from repeating exactly the same motion every day.

Extend shoe life and avoid injury by rotating shoes.

My normal rotation includes five pairs of shoes—two distance shoes, a trail shoe, and two lightweight performance shoes for tempo and interval workouts.

2. Replace Worn Inserts: Another way to increase shoe life is to replace inserts when they lose their cushioning. New inserts are less than $15. That's a great return on investment to extend the life of a $150 shoe. After shopping around, I found inserts that work great for me for less than $10. I bought several pairs.

3. Change Shoes When Finished: Don't wear your running shoes around the house or to run errands. This wears down the cushioning almost as much as running. Change into an old retired pair of running shoes after your run.

4. Repair Worn Outsoles with Shoe Goo: This is an old school trick I learned years ago. When outsoles wear out, you can replace the lost material with Shoe Goo. Some runners are especially hard on the heel because their foot is still going slightly forward upon impact, which quickly scuffs off the heel. Plus, some shoes have very little outsole material. A layer of Shoe Goo every week or so can extend the life of these shoes until the rest of the shoe wears out.

5. Repurpose Old Shoes: Old running shoes can be repurposed as trail shoes, where the need for cushioning is less. Of course, not all road shoes are suitable for trails, but if your shoes are, put in a fresh insert and you're good to go.

Keep Old Shoes as Backup: When your old shoes are worn out, don't toss them. I keep an old pair of shoes in my car in case I get to the workout and find I've forgotten my shoes.

Keep Old Shoes for Diagnostics: Sometimes, a new injury will surface after switching to new shoes. If you can't diagnose the cause of the injury, go for a short run in your old shoes and see if there's any difference. It could help you pinpoint the cause of the new injury. It might be something with your new shoes.

9.   When You Find a Shoe You Like, Stock Up!

A few years ago, I was experiencing severe plantar fasciitis (PF) of the heel. Out of desperation, I tried a new shoe, the Hoka Clifton, which has a radically different heel. It almost immediately solved my PF issue, but it wasn't a good fit for me. Later, I found the Hoka Huaka on clearance and bought a pair. I loved them! Since they were on steep discount, I bought three more pairs. In all, I saved over $300 on those four pairs of shoes.

Bonus Tip: It's not uncommon to see shoes discounted 50% or more in clearance sales. When I find any of my favorite shoes on steep discount, I stock up!

Bonus Tip: Shoe models often change dramatically from year to year. Veterans moan about finding their "perfect" shoe, only to have it ruined by changes in the next year's model. To prevent this from happening to you, buy more than one pair when you find your favorite shoe on sale.

10. Have Different Shoes for Different Runs

Golfers have different clubs for different lies. Fishermen use different hooks and bait for different fish. Football players change cleats depending on the condition of the field, yet many runners use the same shoe for all their workouts. In fact, many marathoners in my training group use the same shoe in their interval workouts, long runs, trail runs, and races. This is not bad per se, as my friends are Boston qualifiers, but they aren't optimizing their ability to become a better runner by using only one pair of shoes. Here's why.

Trail shoes reduce the risk of injury when trail running. The lower heel reduces the risk of rolling your ankle and discourages severe heel striking, which can result in falls on trails. The more aggressive lug pattern reduces the risk of slipping and falling.

Lightweight performance shoes and racing flats can improve race times. Studies have found that every extra ounce of shoe weight slows your race pace by about 1 second per mile.

My distance shoe weighs 9 ounces, and my race shoe weighs 7 ounces. That saves about six seconds in a 5k race. That might not sound like much, but I won a bronze medal in the Huntsman World Games 5K by only five seconds. Shoe weight matters.

Of course, if your goal is to finish a marathon, then your primary concern is not speed, but avoiding injury. In that case, you can stick with the same shoe. Superlight shoes don't provide as much support as a heavier shoe so that they can lead to more injuries. As the old saying goes, "If it ain't broke, don't fix it."

3

Improving Foot Strike

Years ago, no one talked about running form. You just ran. The belief was that if you had any biomechanical flaws in your form, your body would eliminate these flaws as you ran more miles. This was correct to an extent in that it became a self-fulfilling prophecy. Runners with poor form got injured and dropped out of the sport. Fortunately for readers, I loved running too much to quit, so I persevered through those injuries, eventually changing from severe heel striker to a forefoot strike. In this chapter, I'll share the advantages of this change, so you can decide if transitioning to forefoot strike is right for you.

Understanding foot strike mechanics can help you avoid running injuries and become a better runner. To be sure, there are a lot of other biomechanics involved in great running form: arm swing, core, pelvic tilt, and forward lean, just to name a few, but no single aspect is more important than foot strike.

In Chapter 16 "12 Tips to Unlock Free Speed," you'll learn several tips to improve your running form. Until then, let's look at how form changes can help reduce running injuries.

11.   Avoid Injuries: Learn Proper Foot Biomechanics

The human foot—as well as the foot of all running mammals without hooves—is designed to land on the ball of the foot, but 95% of runners are heel strikers. Unfortunately, heel striking can create many problems.

When the foot strikes hard on the heel, there are two separate impacts a few milliseconds apart. On the first impact, the force travels through the heel bone, shins, and hip joints. Over time this first impact can create heel spurs, shin splints, stress fractures, and hip pointers. As bad as this sounds, the second impact is even worse.

After the heel hits, the foot slams forward to land hard on the forefoot a few milliseconds later. This second impact is slightly greater in terms of force, but the real villain is the speed of this second impact. It happens so fast that it creates massive pressure on the arch (plantar fascia). This flattens the arch, pronates the foot, and tilts the ankle inwards. This, in turn, twists the Achilles tendon, the shin, and the kneecap.

Flattening of the arch can cause plantar fasciitis. The twisting motion stresses the Achilles, twists the tibia while also compressing it, and forces the knee to the inside, putting stress on the ACL and the meniscus. The result of this flattening and twisting force can be plantar fasciitis, Achilles tendinitis, shin splints, stress fractures, runners knee, IT band syndrome, and more.

On the other hand, if the foot lands on the forefoot or almost simultaneously on the heel and forefoot, the foot pronates less and the twisting forces are significantly reduced. Simultaneously, the forefoot splays to distribute the force of the impact over a longer time. This allows the impact to be disbursed throughout the leg muscles (which act as shock absorbers) and the tendons (which act like springs to capture rebound energy for the push off).

To understand how a slower impact dissipates impact forces, imagine hitting your finger with a hammer. It hurts a lot. Now imagine hitting your finger very slowly with the same hammer. It doesn't hurt at all. The weight of the hammer hasn't changed. The duration of the impact has been spread out over more time. This is similar to what happens in forefoot versus heel striking.

Severe heel striking increases risk of almost all common running injuries.

If forefoot strike makes runners less injury prone, why are 95% of runners heel strikers? Why do traditional running shoes have a 10-12 mm heel-to-toe drop to encourage heel strike?

The reason is that when developing the modern running shoe, early researchers discovered when runners got tired, they compensated by overstriding and landing on their heels. By adding more heel cushion, they found that runners could routinely land on their heels, increasing the amount of time they could run after getting fatigued.

They also discovered that at slow speed, heel striking is as efficient or even more efficient than forefoot striking.

For shorter runners, the point at which forefoot striking becomes more efficient is around 7 minutes per mile. For taller runners, it's around 6 minutes per mile or faster.

Considering that the overwhelming number of runners run slower than 7 minutes per mile, it's obvious why running shoes are designed to encourage heel striking. Even at the prestigious Boston Marathon, less than 1% of finishers ran faster than a 6-minute mile pace.

Ironically, this means that the stability shoe you thought was designed to prevent injuries by stopping pronation actually exacerbates the problem. It encourages you to land on your heel!

12. Should You Switch to Forefoot Strike?

If forefoot strike is more efficient at speed and reduces the risk of injury, should you switch from heel strike to forefoot strike? Not necessarily. Here's how to decide.

a. Have you always been injury free and have no plans to race faster than a 7 minute per mile pace? If so, there's no reason to change.

b. Do you want to race significantly faster than 7 minutes per mile? Or, are you plagued by one or more of the injuries that are exacerbated by heel strike? In either case, you should consider transitioning to forefoot or a very light heel strike.

Case study: I was a severe heel striker until 2002. I would land with my foot dorsiflexed, toe pointing up in the air, and knee fully extended. As a result, I developed severe knee problems that prevented me from running more than 3 miles without knee supports.

Out of desperation, I decided to change from heel to forefoot strike. Because there was very little advice back then on how to change foot strike, it took me nearly nine months to transition. (You should be able to transition in half that time using the tips in this book.) Once I finally transitioned to forefoot, my knee problems disappeared, and I became a faster runner. I can run 200m at age 70 almost as fast as I did at age 50!

However, everything I did was geared towards making me faster at distances of 200 to 5,000 meters. If your race distance is the marathon or half marathon and you're not constantly injured, there may be no need to change your foot strike. You will be as efficient or even more efficient as a heel striker. Just avoid severe heel striking.

13. Avoid Barefoot Running

For a while, barefoot running was a major fad. Today you'll still find a few runners who swear by its benefits. Will barefoot running make you a better runner? The answer is probably no, but there is one exception. Here's a quick primer on barefoot running.

Advocates correctly point out that humans have evolved for tens of thousands of years to run barefoot. That's true, but these barefoot hominids didn't run on asphalt, which is far harder than dirt. Plus, that's not how *you* evolved. Chances are you have been wearing shoes since you were about three years old. As a result, your foot bones and ligaments are far weaker than if you had gone barefoot all your life. This creates problems when runners attempt to run barefoot too far or too soon on muscles unaccustomed to these new stresses. Podiatrists report a very high incident of stress fractures of the foot in barefoot runners.

Barefoot running increases the risk of some foot injuries.

---

14. Barefoot Running Doesn't Cure Injuries

If barefoot running can cause injuries, why do advocates swear that barefoot running cured their injuries?

The reason is that barefoot running dramatically changes running form.

Barefoot running itself doesn't cure injuries. It's the dramatic shift in running form.

Barefoot running makes it impossible to heel strike, so the foot is forced to land more midfoot or forefoot. This dramatically changes how impact forces are transferred throughout the lower body. In most cases, the actual cure was not barefoot running. It was the dramatic change in running form.

Although I am not a proponent of barefoot running, I routinely do barefoot running drills. After a track workout, I'll take off my shoes and do several strides back and forth on the football field. My feet have a warm glow after I finish these strides that feels like a foot massage. These barefoot drills help strengthen my feet to prevent future foot injuries. Many elite masters runners also do barefoot drills before or after their workout.

Nonetheless, my philosophy is "whatever works for you." If you have recurring chronic injuries *and* these injuries don't respond to the treatments suggested in the injury chapter of this book, then you might want to try barefoot running.

15.   The Limitations of Heel Striking

There is nothing wrong with a light heel strike for most recreational runners. However, heel striking has three major limitations. 1. Even light heel strikers will land harder on their heels as they get fatigued, and severe heel striking increases injury risk. 2. Heel strikers are at a disadvantage at paces faster than 6 minutes/mile. 3. Heel striking puts you at risk of being outkicked at the end of a race. If any of these criteria affect you, then you should consider the following drills to lessen your heel strike. The competition chapter describes some of these drills in more detail, but here's how to begin.

16.   Transitioning to Forefoot Strike

It's almost impossible to heel strike when running barefoot. Artificial turf or well-groomed grass will cushion the shock and make the following drill easier. Stand barefoot on a grass or turf football field. Without bending at the waist, lean forward until you feel yourself falling forward. Then, run with easy strides back and forth on the field as you focus on how the barefoot landing feels.

You'll become consciously aware you are landing on your forefoot, not the heel. You'll be taking somewhat faster, more compact strides and running with a slight forward lean. The lean might not be obvious to you, but you can confirm it exists by having someone videotape you while doing this drill. It's not a bend at the waist; the entire body should lean forward. Your foot tendons and muscles will be unaccustomed to barefoot running so don't do more than 4 to 6 strides the first time out.

After a few strides, immediately put on your shoes and attempt to recreate that same form on the track. This is not about speed, so there's no need to run fast. Because you are wearing traditional running shoes with a heel lift, you might still heel strike, but it will be a softer heel strike.

In the competition chapter, you'll learn several drills that will ease your transition to forefoot strike. The common denominator of these drills is that they promote a slight forward lean, which promotes landing more on the forefoot.

Warning: Once you get the hang of running on the forefoot, don't make the mistake of going out for a ten-mile run. It will take months for your tendons and muscles to get strong enough to handle this new running form without injury. Gradually increase the distance of your forefoot runs over time.

17   Consider a Low Heel-to-toe Drop Shoe

If you watch a slow-motion video of the foot strike of elite runners, you'll notice their feet are often nearly parallel to the ground before foot strike. If the shoe has a higher heel, the heel might strike first, but if the shoe has no heel lift, the forefoot might touch first. Even a tiny amount of heel lift can affect how the foot hits the ground.

If you decide to convert to forefoot strike, your transition will go faster if you run in a shoe with a low heel-to-toe drop. The higher the heel, the more difficult it becomes to land on the forefoot.

Traditional running shoes have a heel-to-toe drop of 10 mm, but shoes with a 4-6 mm drop allow for a less pronounced heel strike. In fact, I've been a forefoot striker for so long that I can no longer run in traditional 10 mm heel-to-toe drop shoes.

Some modern running shoes have zero heel lift, so the position of the foot upon landing is somewhat similar to running barefoot. I've tried zero heel lift shoes, but I can't run in them. For me, the sweet spot is about 4 mm of heel lift. You'll have to determine what works best for you.

One problem you will encounter when looking for low-heeled shoes is that many running shoes neglect forefoot cushioning. You'll probably experience a sore forefoot in the first few weeks as you transition. Running on a soft surface can alleviate this problem.

18.   Consider Rocker Sole Shoes

Shoes with a curved or rocker sole can also ease your transition into forefoot or lighter heel strike running. In rocker soled shoes, the toe and heel curve upwards from the midfoot of the shoe. In a side photo of the shoe, the heel and toe will be elevated, with only the midfoot touching the ground. If you push down on the toe of the shoe and then release, the shoe will rock back and forth—hence the moniker "rocker sole."

The upward curve in the heel combined with the low heel-to-toe drop creates a rolling action upon landing rather than the sudden, jarring impact of traditional shoes. Several companies make rocker sole shoes, but I only have firsthand experience with two—Hoka and Skechers.

I've owned several models of these two brands. The fit and feel are quite different from one model to the other, so don't give up if the first model you try doesn't feel right. The Skechers are a better fit for me in the toebox, but I prefer Hokas once I get them modified for my foot. You'll learn more about shoe modification in an upcoming chapter.

By the way, you aren't limited to these brands. The success of Hokas has led other manufacturers to make shoes with variations of the rocker sole design. In a recent visit to a running store, I saw four other brands with models that had a pronounced upward curve in the heel.

These rocker heeled shoes have saved the careers of many older runners. If you're experiencing foot problems, you should give them a try.

4

How to Avoid Injuries

Only a very few people are blessed with the perfect genetics to run without injury. I'm not one of those runners. Most likely, you aren't either. According to the American College of Sports Medicine Journal, 50-70% of runners training for their first marathon drop out before the race due to injury. According to the SMART Institute of the University of South Florida, the average runner will miss 5-10% of their workouts due to injury and novice runners are significantly more likely to be injured than veteran runners.

At least once a year, most runners will experience an injury lasting long enough to adversely impact their training program. Thus, it's extremely important to learn how to identify, treat, and prevent common running injuries.

19. Analyze Your Injuries

When runners complain about their latest injury, I always ask, "What caused it?" I usually get a blank stare, followed by, "Um... running?" Well, sure, but what specifically caused it? Many runners don't have a clue.

Recurring injuries can sabotage your running goals, so when you get injured, it's important to figure out what caused the injury. Then, you can take steps to ensure that it doesn't happen again. Simple—yet many runners don't follow this advice.

When a debilitating injury occurs, runners should ask themselves *where exactly* is the pain? What *caused* this injury? What was I doing when it occurred? What was different in my routine that might have caused this injury? If the injury doesn't seem to have a cause related to your most recent run, look further into the past to see if the injury occurred earlier.

When an injury occurs, ask, "What caused it?"
Use that knowledge to prevent it in the future.

For example, at a recent track meet, I felt a pain in my quadriceps during my warm-up routine. I carefully went through this list of questions and could identify no apparent cause. When I looked further into the past, I remembered that I had done barbell squats a couple of days earlier. I vaguely recalled a twinge at the time, but I didn't think anything of it. Thus, running was not the cause of the problem; running had merely exacerbated a minor injury caused by weightlifting.

I had gone to the meet in great shape with a goal of setting a time that would position me high in the national rankings. I kept warming up easily. The pain was not debilitating enough to prevent me from racing. I could run, but should I?

For me, the decision was easy. I scratched out of the race, took a few days off, and avoided lifting since that was the cause of the injury. In a few days, the injury resolved itself. If I had not analyzed the cause, I would have taken time off running but continued to lift, reinjuring the quad and causing even more time off.

It was the right move, yet only very experienced runners have the discipline to do this. Why? More to the point, why are decisions like this so difficult for some runners and yet so easy for me? I call this process "pre-deciding." You'll learn how to do it in Chapter 8.

20. Learn the Difference between Pain and Injury

Pain is something you learn to control as a runner. If you run hard enough and long enough, there's going to be some discomfort. With experience, you can learn how to "run through" minor discomforts of training and racing. Injuries, on the other hand, are quite different.

With an injury, it's important to immediately differentiate between a minor pain and an injury. Perhaps the easiest way to tell if something is an actual injury is to ask yourself whether the pain is symmetrical. For example, if both calves are sore, it's most likely an overuse injury that will go away with time. If only one calf is sore, it's most likely an injury. (An exception to this rule is shin splints, which will be discussed later.)

Injuries are usually asymmetrical.

The best approach with a sharp or sudden onset pain is to slow the pace and see if it goes away. If it doesn't, then you should stop and walk for a few minutes. On the grand scheme of things, those few minutes of walking are not going to impact your training. If the pain doesn't return when you start running again, you're good to go. But if the pain does return, it's probably best to abort the workout and walk home.

Chances are very good that you'll be able to return to normal within a day or so. If you keep running, the injury could get worse—much worse.

21. STOP if You Get Injured!

How many times have you heard the following lament from another runner? "I had just reached mile 2 of my 12-mile run when I felt this shooting pain. It felt like a knife in my knee"—we know how this complaint ends—"so I hobbled to finish my 12-mile run. The next day, my knee was really swollen. It's been two weeks, and I still can't run!"

Too many runners try to push through a minor injury, and as a result, it becomes a major injury that results in losing weeks of valuable training time. I have heard variations of this story dozens of times. Every time, it makes me wince.

If you feel an unusual pain, slow or stop running to assess it. You can prevent minor injuries from becoming major ones.

As we get older and more experienced, we should learn from our mistakes. Yet some runners seemingly never learn this one critical lesson—when you feel an unusual pain, you should slow or stop completely to check it out. If you're lucky, you can catch a minor injury before it becomes serious.

A good example is the quadriceps injury I mentioned a couple of pages back. Aggravating that minor injury could have caused weeks of lost training and prevented me from reaching my primary goals of racing later in the summer.

A few years ago, I went out for a 10-mile run with the Nashville Striders. It was a very social event with over a hundred runners, so I was enjoying running with friends. About three miles in, I felt a sharp pain in my foot. I walked a few steps and tried to run, but the pain returned.

Have you ever been in this position? If so, what would you do?

For me, it the decision was easy. From that point on, my objective completely shifted from enjoying a long run with friends to avoiding a serious injury.

I let everyone else go on and started limping back. It took me over an hour to cover three miles back to my car, but that was very useful time. During that hour, I analyzed the situation to determine the cause of the injury.

The route was new to me and had an unusually steep camber (tilt to the side). The camber had put more pressure on an old foot injury. My foot could handle it for 2 miles, but 3 miles was apparently too much. By identifying the cause, I was able to ensure that I wouldn't repeat that same mistake in the future.

The good news is that the next day, I was able to return to my normal training schedule.

In some areas of life, we are very good at shifting priorities instantly. When a mom hears her child cry in real pain, she immediately drops what she is doing to attend to the child, but when we are personally at risk, we sometimes fail to react as wisely as we should.

A good analogy is a flat tire while going to an important meeting. We see stories in the news all the time where motorists are killed on the side of the road while changing a tire. Sadly, these tragedies often occur because the victim was unable to shift priorities quickly when the flat tire occurred.

If your car breaks down on the side of the road, your immediate priority becomes getting to a safe place. Everything else, including getting to that important meeting, becomes secondary. It's the same with running. When injuries occur, everything else becomes secondary to reducing the risk of further injury.

Finishing a workout today is never more important than running injury-free tomorrow.

The endorphins we get from running can distract us from potentially serious injuries in the early stages. Always maintain awareness of any unusual pains. *There is nothing to be gained by hobbling through miles of a training run with an injury.* Not only can you make the injury worse, but you might also injure something else because you're favoring the injured area.

The best approach is to slow or walk when a new pain occurs. If the pain returns when you try to run again, abort the workout.

It requires more courage to abort a workout than to limp through it.

If I were giving a speech, I'd clap my hands right now to get everyone's attention. It requires more courage to abort a workout than to limp through it. *Finishing a run today is never as important as being able to run injury free tomorrow.*

22. Avoiding Injuries if You are Age 50+

Avoiding injury becomes increasingly important after age 50. As a rule of thumb for younger runners, every week lost to injury takes about two weeks of training to get back to your preinjury level of fitness. That means if you're injured for a month, it takes two months to get back to the same level of fitness you had before the injury.

Injuries take longer to heal as we age, so avoiding injury becomes critically important for older runners.

That rule of thumb begins to change dramatically somewhere between ages 50 and 60. If you lose a month of training at age 50, it might take 3 to 4 months to get back to your preinjury level of performance. If you lose a month of training after age 60, *you might never recover to that preinjury level of fitness.*

With that in mind, here's how to reduce your risk of injury.

- When you feel an unusual pain, slow down or walk to assess it. If the pain continues, abort the workout. If you catch it soon enough, chances are you'll be fine the next day.

- Take two pairs of shoes to workouts. Minor foot injuries can sometimes be alleviated by simply changing shoes.

- Make your own orthotics—explained in Chapter 6.

- Learn how to tape your arch, heel, and ankle—explained in an upcoming chapter—for extra support while recovering from minor injuries.

- Avoid terrain that is problematic for you. In my case, I avoid steeply cambered roads whenever possible.

- Avoid high-risk cross training. (More detail on this later.)

23. Cut Your Injury Risk by Half!

Studies show that half of running injuries are recurrences of old injuries. If you identify the cause of each new injury, you can then take steps to prevent that injury in the future.

---

*Simply by identifying the cause of each injury,
you can cut your future injuries by half!*

Still, many runners have chronic problems with blisters, black toenails, shin splints, runners knee, and more. I *never* get these injuries. In the next two chapters, you'll learn how to banish them forever.

5

Preventing Common Running Injuries

This publication contains the opinions and ideas of its author. It is sold with the understanding that the author and publisher are not engaged in rendering medical, health, or any other kind of personal professional services in the book. The reader should consult his or her medical, health, or other competent professional before adopting any of the suggestions in this book or in drawing inferences from it. The author and publisher specifically disclaim all responsibility for any liability, loss, or risk, personal or otherwise, that is incurred as a consequence, directly or indirectly, of the use and application of any of the contents of this book.

In 40 years of running, I've experienced more injuries than I can count. In fact, looking back over the past 20 years in my running journal, I've never been able to run longer than nine months without a significant injury. Sometimes, I marvel that I'm still running, much less able to remain competitive.

The silver lining to all those injuries is that they gave me a wealth of experience in treating and preventing running injuries. In this chapter, I'll share what I've learned with the hope that this knowledge will speed your recovery from the injuries that are bound to occur eventually when your feet hit the pavement 10,000 times every hour in our favorite sport.

This could be the most valuable chapter in this book, but first, a word of caution. I'm not a doctor. Plus, I can't even see your injury. Symptoms can appear to be one injury, but the real injury might be something else. As a result, my suggestions might not work for you. See a medical professional if the problem persists.

If ever there was a case where an ounce of prevention is worth a pound of cure, it's in preventing common running injuries. Seeing a physical therapist for several weeks can be expensive, not to mention the loss of training time, so it behooves every runner to take proactive steps to avoid injuries. When injuries inevitably do occur, you need to treat them quickly so you can return to running as soon as possible.

Your running shoes are one of the most likely suspects for running injuries because that's where all the impact starts. Let's begin by reassessing the misconceptions most runners have about shoes.

24. Be Willing to Modify Your Shoes

While some runners can find a shoe that's almost a perfect fit, it's not the case for most of us. For millions of runners, the sad truth is the perfect shoe doesn't exist.

Don't get me wrong; it's still a good idea to get the best fit possible when buying shoes, but the reality is even the best shoe may not be perfect for your unique foot and biomechanics.

As a result, you may need to modify your shoes to improve the fit. We buy suits anticipating they will need to be tailored, yet runners take new shoes out of the box and expect them to fit perfectly for hundreds of miles. That doesn't make sense.

Imagine buying a new car and then driving it without adjusting the seat and mirrors. You'd never do that. Yet those same people would take their running shoes out of the box and run in them with no adjustments at all. It's a testament to the miraculous adaptability of the human body that running injuries aren't even more prevalent.

Obviously, you should start with the best shoe fit you can find, but you should also be willing to modify your shoes to prevent or treat your running injuries. Sometimes the "perfect" shoe can cause one little nagging problem, yet you love it in every other respect. Maybe you can salvage it using one or more of the modifications in this chapter.

25. But It Can't Be My Shoes!

Some runners may scoff at the idea their shoes could be a problem. "It can't be my shoes! I've worn the same shoes for ten years." Still, it's possible your shoes are contributing to your current injury. Here's why.

- **Worn Shoes.** As shoes wear out, they lose cushioning and lack the stability of new shoes.

- **New Model.** Shoes can change dramatically from one model year to the next, which can change the fit of the shoe.

- **You Change.** Over the years, you change due to aging and the accumulation of miles. While the shoe might not have caused the initial injury, they may lack sufficient support to prevent the injury from getting worse.

- **All of the Above.** Perhaps it's not one of these reasons, but a combination of them all that can cause your tried and true shoe model to contribute to injuries.

26.   Pain Under the Eyelets

Shoes can sometimes cause painful bruising immediately under the eyelets—either because the lacing is too tight or the eyelet is reinforced with a plastic ring that pushes against the top of the foot. In either case, the solution is easy. Simply skip that eyelet when lacing the shoes. Another approach is to create a new eyelet by punching a hole nearby with a nail or drill. An even better long-term prevention approach is to use elastic laces, which are described in more detail later in this chapter.

27.   Blisters on the Little Toe

Shoes that are too narrow can lead to blisters on the little toe or between the toes from being squeezed together. There are several possible solutions to fix this. The best approach is to buy shoes that are wider in the toe box or a half size larger, but if the shoe is great in all other ways, you have some additional options.

The easiest approach is to wear thinner socks, which effectively makes the toe box wider. Next, you can skip the bottom set of eyelets nearest the toes to let the toe box stretch more. I routinely take both these steps.

That might be enough for you. But if not, the next step is to remove the outer layer of decorative overlay covering the side of the little toe. To do this, take a box cutter and carefully cut the threads holding the leather to the mesh, peel it back from the mesh, and then cut off this little strip of leather. The underlying mesh will then be free to stretch more.

If the shoe still feels snug, remove the ½ inch-or-so wide horizontal strip of leather that runs along the outside of the shoe on the side adjacent to the little toe. Not all shoes have this, but if yours do, you can remove it. It won't affect the structural integrity of the shoe.

When buying new shoes, be aware of the fit in the toe box. If you can feel the toe box pressing against your little toe when you're trying on the shoe, it's probably going to cause blisters because your feet will swell as you run. You need to look for a different shoe or a half size larger.

Until the blister heals, cover it with a waterproof Band-Aid. I usually peel the pad off the Band-Aid, so the material is a little thinner. After all, if the shoe is too narrow, you're just making it worse by adding the padding of a Band-Aid in that spot.

28. Black Toenails

Black toenails are caused when toenails rub against the top or the front of the toe box. Eventually, the nail gets so bruised that it gets black and falls off. The most common cause is shoes that are too small. This is especially true for women who tend to buy their shoes a little too small. In this case, the solution is easy—buy a half size larger shoe or a shoe with a bigger toe box.

Orthotics can also cause black toenail because they are sometimes thicker in the forefoot, pushing the toes into the roof of the toe box. Again, the solution is to buy a bigger shoe with a taller toe box.

Less often, black toenails can be caused by a shoe that is too big. The foot slides forward inside the shoe with each step and the toenail jams against the front of the toe box. This is common in downhill running and heel strikers. Severe heel striking is a braking action, which momentarily causes the foot to slide forward in the shoe. In this case, the solution is elastic lacing or butterfly lacing, both of which we'll discuss in this chapter.

Unfortunately, some runners have toenails that point up, so they can snag against the toe box with each step. There isn't a great solution for this. Your best bet would be to trim your toenails often and wear shoes without a toe box cover—a leather strip around the front of the shoe—or a shoe with a tall toe box.

29. Morton's Neuroma

Morton's Neuroma is a nasty injury that can put you on crutches or have you limping for weeks. It's an inflammation around the bones of the ball of the foot. Often, the cause is a shoe that is too narrow in the toe box. This squeezes the bones of the foot together, causing inflammation and swelling because the bones rub together with each step.

Since this happens about 10,000 times in an hour run, it's a wonder this problem isn't more common, but there are ways to fix it. The logical step is to buy a half-size larger shoe or a shoe with a wider toe box. That's definitely what you should do in the future, but there may be ways to salvage your existing shoes.

A too-narrow toe box can cause Morton's Neuroma.

Several solutions for Morton's Neuroma are the same as for little toe blisters. First, make your forefoot smaller by wearing a thinner sock. It's hard to find super thin men's socks, but they're easy to find in the women's department. They come in neutral colors and aren't any thicker than a T-shirt. A women's large fits my size 9½ foot.

Thinner socks will help, but they might not be enough by themselves. So, the next step is to make the forefoot of the shoe wider. First, replace the existing insert with a thinner insert from another pair of shoes. Then, re-lace the shoes, skipping the bottom set of eyelets nearest the toes.

Taken together, these three steps—thinner socks, a thinner insert, and skipping the bottom eyelets—should be enough, but if it doesn't resolve the problem, you can make even more room by modifying the shoe itself.

Many running shoes have a protective leather strip that runs from the bottom eyelets down the outside of each shoe towards the little toe. They might also have a leather strip that runs around the front of the toe box ending just past the little toe. This material doesn't stretch and contributes to the tightness of the shoe, but it can be removed. Cut the stitching carefully along this leather covering. Then cut the strips off the shoe in the area of the little toe. There will be mesh underneath, so cut carefully to leave the mesh intact and in place.

If this doesn't work, there's one final step you can try. Most shoes have a reinforcing piece of leather where the tongue is attached to the toe box. Cut through that material making a vertical slit about one inch long going towards the toe of the shoe. You should cut through the underlying mesh as well. When finished, you'll have a slit about a half inch into the tongue and about a half inch past the tongue going towards the toe of the shoe.

This slit will be almost invisible with the shoe off, but when you put the shoe on, it will bulge open a bit. The reason it bulges open is that your shoe is too narrow. Remember, that's been the problem all along, so next time, buy a half size larger or a different shoe with a wider toe box.

If these modifications don't resolve the problem, you should throw these shoes away. Even if you stop running until it heals, the shoe might cause the same problem when you start running again. You shouldn't even keep them for walking.

Bonus Tip: During rehab, it's important that your toes have room to splay out, so you may need wider casual shoes to wear when you're not running. This is important because once you get Morton's Neuroma, you're prone to getting it again.

30. Butterfly or Heel Lock Lacing

Some runners develop blisters or calluses because their shoes are too wide in the heel, which causes the heel to slide up and down or the foot to slide back and forth in the shoe. One way to solve this problem is butterfly lacing, also called heel lock lacing. If you're using it, remove the laces from the top eyelet closest to your ankle. (Shoes typically come with this eyelet unlaced.) Starting with the second eyelet from the top, insert the lace into the top eyelet on the same side of the shoe. Repeat on the other side, but don't pull the laces tight. This will form a loop between the top eyelet and the eyelet immediately below it. Run the left lace end through the loop on the right side. Reverse this process with the right shoelace. Then, pull the laces tight. This pulls the heel cup of the shoe forward and results in a snug, slip-free fit.

Butterfly lacing can help prevent black toenail if your foot is slipping forward in the shoe upon heel strike.

I used butterfly lacing for years until I found an even better approach—elastic laces. You'll read about them soon, but first, let's look a little closer at heel blisters.

31. Blisters from Heel Slippage

If your heel is very narrow, butterfly lacing might not be enough to prevent heel blisters. Obviously, you would be better off buying a narrower shoe, but the following steps might salvage a shoe that you love in all other respects.

- Wear thicker socks.

- Use elastic laces combined with butterfly lacing. How to make your own elastic laces is explained later in this chapter. Elastic laces let you pull the laces tighter to keep the heel in place without the risk of bruising the top of your foot, which can happen with regular laces.

- Punch a new set of eyelets about 3/4 inch closer to the heel of the shoe than the top set of eyelets. You can use a nail or cordless drill to make the hole. Skip the original top set of eyelets and use this new set of eyelets for butterfly lacing. This should really secure the heel into the shoe and stop any slipping. Elastic laces work better for this, but you can try it with regular laces first. But beware, you can bruise the top of your foot where the laces cross doing this with regular laces.

- As a last resort, you can make the heel collar narrower. About 3" from the heel on the inside of the shoe, you'll see where the heel collar material is sewn into the front material. Cut a piece of crafts felt about 2" wide and 6" long, put it into the shoe, and curve it around the heel, so it forms another layer of heel collar material. Carefully put on the shoe so as not to move the felt and do a short test run. In addition to a snug fit in the heel, this will shove your foot forward in the shoe almost as if it were a half size smaller. If you're okay with this shorter feel, trim the felt to fit and use spray glue to hold it in place.

32. Top of Foot Bruising

You might wonder, how can you possibly get a bruise on the top of the foot? The problem is the laces are too tight. This is like the eyelet bruising discussed earlier, but it tends to occur where the laces cross rather than under the eyelets.

This problem is more common among runners who have high arches or wear orthotics, which pushes the top of the foot higher than normal. Or, the runner could just be lacing the shoe too tightly. Fortunately, there are two fixes for this problem.

The first solution is to skip the eyelet where the lacing is pressing against the foot and causing pain. Just lace from one eyelet to the eyelet directly above it before continuing to cross the laces. You can lace most running shoes adequately using only half the eyelets provided anyway. Not lacing over the pressure point eliminates the pain instantly. Try it— you'll be amazed that you didn't think of it yourself.

My current running shoe has seven sets of eyelets. I only use four on the left shoe and five on the right. Unless you have a narrow foot, you simply don't need to use all those eyelets.

The second solution is to replace the cloth laces with elastic laces.

33. Elastic Laces Fix a Major Flaw in Running Shoes

Every pair of running shoes has one major flaw—the laces. In fact, since Bill Bowerman first started making shoes with his waffle iron back in the 60s and created the company that would eventually become Nike, shoelaces haven't changed very much.

You might be one of the lucky runners who has never experienced a shoelace-related injury, but take it from someone who has, traditional shoelaces can cause injuries. With each step, your foot expands when it impacts the ground. Or, more precisely, it attempts to expand.

Traditional laces prevent this expansion, which can lead to a myriad of foot injuries. On the other hand, with elastic laces, you can see the laces stretch upon impact as the foot expands naturally upon landing.

In turn, this lessens the impact directly under the eyelet and where the laces cross. Elastic laces also allow tighter lacing to prevent the foot from sliding inside the shoe, which can cause calluses, blisters, or black toenail.

Elastic laces alleviate many common foot injuries—black toenail, Morton's Neuroma, bruising under laces and eyelets, blisters, and more.

Some runners attempt to solve these problems by keeping their shoelaces very loose, but this creates its own set of problems as the foot moves inside the shoe—black toenail, blisters, and the risk of rolling your ankle. Let's look at how several common problems can be eliminated with elastic laces.

- **Morton's Neuroma.** Tight lacing prevents the foot from expanding when it hits the ground. This can cause bruising between the bones of the forefoot (Morton's Neuroma).

- **Bruises on top of the foot.** The same tight lacing can cause bruising under the eyelets of the shoe or where the laces cross. Elastic lacing allows the laces to stretch so the foot can flex, preventing these injuries.

- **Black toenail.** Conversely, tying the shoe too loose can let the foot slide inside the shoe, jamming the toes against the toe box and causing black toenail.

- **Blisters.** Loose lacing also can cause blisters as the foot slides inside the shoe.

- **Ankle injury.** The foot sliding in the shoe increases the risk of rolling your ankle. Elastic laces snug the foot in place inside the shoe, preventing the sliding that can cause black toenail, blisters, and rolled ankles.

- **Ease of putting on/taking off.** Elastic lacing makes shoes as easy to put on and take off as bedroom slippers.

Traditional laces can also come untied at the worst times. If you haven't experienced an untied shoelace in a race, you aren't racing much, or you've been extremely lucky. If a shoe comes untied in a group run, stopping to tie it again can put you a half minute behind your training partners. Then you have to struggle for miles to catch up.

Elastic laces don't become untied because they aren't tied to begin with. They're held in place by a cord lock. To adjust the tightness, you give the cord a quick tug and slip the cord lock tighter.

You can double knot your traditional laces to prevent them from becoming untied, but that can create more problems. First, you can forget to do it. Second, it takes more time, especially to remove the double knot. Third, adjusting the tightness after you've tied the double knot is a hassle.

Case study: I wear my shoes snug to prevent injuries. If my shoes are too loose or too tight with traditional laces, adjusting the laces for both shoes can take a minute. With elastic laces, I can tighten or loosen the laces in less than five seconds per shoe.

At your next race, look at the laces of other runners. Almost no one is wearing elastic laces, yet this is one of the easiest steps you can take to prevent shoe-related injuries.

With elastic laces, shoes never come untied!

---

34. How to Make Elastic Laces

Although you can buy elastic laces, I prefer to make my own using one-eighth inch shock cord and a cord lock. Shock cord is inexpensive and readily available on eBay and other online vendors. Cut a length of shock cord about three feet long. Melt the ends with a match so they won't fray. Remove the old laces and push the ends of the shock cord through the eyelets.

You may have to widen the eyelets by pushing a ballpoint pen or a nail through the existing eyelet. If the eyelets are hard plastic, you can use a drill to make them wider. Once threaded through all the eyelets, put on the cord lock and pull it tight to fit the shoe to your foot. When tight, there should be about 4-5 inches of cord sticking out above the cord lock. If it's longer, trim it off and melt the ends again so it won't fray. Then, tie a knot at the end of the shock cord so the laces can't inadvertently slip through the cord lock when you take off your shoes.

You can try elastic laces for free. Just cut the elastic cord and cord locks off the hood or waistline of an unused winter coat. It stretches, so it doesn't take much cord. There should be enough for a pair of shoes.

Once you prove to yourself that shock cord laces are the greatest thing to running since the invention of the shoe, you can buy enough shock cord and cord locks online to make a dozen or so elastic laces for about a dollar a pair. When your buddies comment on your elastic laces, you can give them one of your "spare" pairs. They'll be so grateful that they'll offer to buy you a beer.

Once you make a set of elastic laces, you can transfer them to new shoes when your old shoes wear out. I've used the same set of elastic laces for years.

Improve your running shoes with elastic laces!

The first thing I do when buying new shoes is remove the factory laces and install shock cord laces.

Of course, you can buy elastic laces in running stores for $4 to $8, but there is one shortcoming to commercial elastic laces. They're made from thinner shock cord so they'll easily fit through the eyelets of all running shoes. If you prefer to keep your laces really snug as I do, these thinner laces need to be pulled so tight that they lose most of their elasticity. That negates the stretchiness and injury prevention advantages of the thicker 1/8-inch shock cord.

35. Blisters on the Arch

If you get blisters on the arch, the first step is to determine exactly where the blister is occurring in relation to the inside parts of your shoe. If the blister is on the bottom of your foot, the culprit might be your socks. If you are wearing thick socks that don't fit tightly across the arch, your foot could be sliding within the sock. The solution is to wear a tighter sock with compression material across the arch and to use elastic laces.

If the blister is where the side wall of the shoe meets the insert, the insert might be pinching the foot where the edge of the insert meets the side wall. The shoe needs some protective material here, so remove the insert and tape a piece of felt under the arch of the insert, extending it an inch or so past the edge of the insert adjacent to the blister. The felt should now extend up the inside of the shoe, covering the inner material of the shoe that was causing the blister.

On rare occasions, a design flaw can cause blisters. The 2016 Hoka Clayton had a stiff upper material that caused blisters just above the insert at the inside edge of the arch. I owned this shoe and didn't have this problem, but if I had, I would have simply cut out the offending area.

36. Bruised Ankle Bone

Sometimes, the heel collar can be too high, which bounces against the ankle bone with each stride, eventually resulting in a nagging ankle bruise. The best way to avoid this is to buy shoes with a lower heel collar, but you might not notice the problem until you've worn the shoe several times. Or, you like the shoes, except for this one problem. Fortunately, the fix is easy. Simply add a couple of layers of crafts felt under the insert in the heel area. This will lift the foot enough that the ankle bone isn't striking the heel collar. If you don't have crafts felt, any material will do, like a piece of an old T-shirt.

If the added material raises your heel uncomfortably high, there's another solution. Using scissors, cut off the sides of the heel collar, so they are a half-inch lower. Surprisingly, once you put the shoe on, this shoe surgery will become virtually invisible.

37. Achilles Tendonitis

Achilles tendonitis is a serious injury. It took me two years to recover the first time. The second time was only a few weeks because I caught it early and immediately stopped running. I then went into aggressive treatment mode because the Huntsman World Games were only six weeks away.

I took two weeks off. I used Epsom Salt soaks in hot water. I didn't ice the injury because there was no swelling. (Icing is only beneficial if there is swelling with the injury or immediately after the injury to prevent swelling.) I also used an inferential TENS unit and a liniment to speed blood flow to the area. You'll learn more about these techniques in Chapter 8.

Once the pain was gone, I resumed slow running after taping the Achilles with KT tape starting in front of the heel, then going over the heel directly up the Achilles, and stopping at mid-calf. I pointed my toes down and stretched the KT tape when applying it, so there was a lot of tension provided by the tape as my foot dorsiflexed. I shaved my legs and used alcohol first to make sure the tape would stick. I also added a loop of tape around the calf and over the KT tape to keep it from pulling loose because it was stretched so tight. I taped for another three weeks.

During this time, I avoided hills, sprints, and pushing off—anything that would stretch the Achilles.

Achilles injuries can be serious. Don't try to run through it. Treat this injury as if your entire running career depended on it.

Let me stress that Achilles tendonitis can be a career-ending injury if you don't take it seriously. I stopped running at the first twinge of pain. Had I continued to run, it's very likely that the injury would've gotten worse. Even though I lost nearly six weeks of training, my aggressive rehab approach allowed me to race at the Huntsman World Games, winning two gold and a bronze medal only six weeks after the injury.

38. Hamstring Injuries

Hamstring injuries can be nagging little pains that never seem to heal completely. They get better for a while and then the pain comes back. It's usually not so bad that it keeps you from running completely, but it just never seems to end.

Typically, with hamstring injury runners might take a couple of days off and then attempt to jog a few paces. If there's no pain, they start off on a conservative run. The hamstring is okay for a while, but then out of the blue—ouch!—there's a sudden pain. Depending on the runner's pain threshold—or stubbornness!—they'll either stop or struggle through the workout. In either case, the damage was done on the first "ouch." A strand of muscle tissue was partially re-torn. The next day the hamstring is too sore to run. This process can go on for weeks or even months.

Here's the secret to hamstring injuries. The reason the pain keeps re-occurring is that you are running before the scar tissue has fully healed. The tissue might handle running for a mile or so, but eventually, it re-tears, which forces the healing process to start over from day one.

To treat hamstring injuries, you must limit the range of motion of the hamstring until the scar tissue gets strong enough to handle running again.

The secret to hamstring injuries is to avoid stretching and restrict the range of motion until the scar tissue can heal enough to handle easy running.

Rather than cover this twice, you can read a detailed explanation of stretching for hamstring injuries in tip 54.

39. Shin Splints

The term shin splint is commonly used to describe two different injuries: shin splints and stress fractures of the shin bone. A shin splint is a strain of the soft tissue in front of the shin, whereas a stress fracture is a hairline crack in the bone itself. Although these injuries are related, runners will need a slightly different approach for each one.

Shin splints are more common among beginners and women, but they can also occur as runners increase their weekly mileage. The muscles, ligaments, and bones haven't grown strong enough to handle the extra stress caused by the repetitive impact.

You can sometimes tell the difference between a stress fracture and a shin splint by pressing the shin with your thumb. If there is a sharp pain in one exact location, it may be a stress fracture.

Shin splints in beginners can sometimes be cured by drills, such as eccentric calf raises, toe lifts, heel walks, and other drills to stretch the soft tissue. While rehabbing this injury, runners should reduce the pounding on this injured tissue by running on softer surfaces.

To prevent stress fractures from reoccurring, you will need to change your form. First, become consciously aware of the sound of your foot strike and make it quieter. Runners with a very loud foot strike typically run almost vertically, landing with the knee almost locked and with a pronounced heel strike. This puts stress on the shins. In an upcoming chapter, you'll learn form drills to improve running form and reduce the risk of shin splints and stress fractures.

Rocker Sole Shoes: Different running shoes may help, but they will only address a symptom of the problem, not the actual cause. An exception might be rocker sole shoes, which change how the heel impacts the ground.

40. Rocker Sole Shoes Might Extend Your Career

Three years ago, I had a severe case of plantar fasciitis on the heel of my foot. The pain was so bad that I kept crutches beside the bed to use in the morning until the soreness went away enough to walk. None of my usual plantar fasciitis treatments worked. After months of recovering about 50% and then getting reinjured, I finally solved the problem with dry needling, TENS stimulation, and rocker soled shoes. Dry needling and TENS will be discussed in a later chapter, so what's the deal with these odd-looking shoes?

A rocker sole shoe has a thicker than normal midsole that rounds upward to the heel and the toe box. The result is a shoe that will "rock" back and forth if you set it on a level surface and press down on the toe box.

At present, there are two major brands in the rocker shoe marketplace: Sketchers and Hoka. Several of my running friends had reported that their chronic injuries disappeared when they switched to the Hoka, so I decided to give it a try. These shoes allowed me to return to running with no further problems.

Rocker sole shoes work because the foot touches down slightly ahead of the heel bone just at the beginning of the midfoot, whereas a traditional shoe touches down directly over the heel bone. Second, in a traditional shoe, the heel hits first and then the forefoot slams down hard, creating a potential for a myriad of running injuries.

The rocker soles on Hoka and Skechers shoes allow the foot to roll forward onto the forefoot rather than slam down. As a result, these rocker sole shoes mimic the advantages of a forefoot strike without going through the hassle of retraining yourself to land on the forefoot.

Caveat: There's a considerable difference in feel between the various models of these shoes. You need to try them on before buying to see if they are right for you. Other brands are now making rocker sole shoes, so ask for them at your local running store.

41   Treat the Cause, Not Just the Symptom

If this book was a speech, this is where you would hear me say, "If you only remember one thing about this speech, it should be this."

Regardless of the injury, *be sure to address the cause of the injury and not just the injury itself.* Most injuries will leave a clue as to the cause, but if you can't figure it out on your own, ask other runners or a doctor. You certainly don't want to take several weeks off for an injury, only to have it reoccur.

**If you don't address the cause of the injury,
there's a strong possibility it will occur again.**

In my opinion, this is one of the biggest mistakes injured runners make. They only treat the injury, not the cause of the injury.

It's possible that your injury might have a different cause. If so, these solutions might not work for you.

In closing, let me stress this chapter only addresses the most likely causes for common running injuries and makes recommendations based on that assumption. Remember, I haven't seen your foot, your injury, your running form, your x-rays, your training schedule, or your medical history. I'm not a doctor. Seek help from a medical professional for all running injuries. You should consult a medical, health, or other competent professional before adopting any of the suggestions in this book or in drawing inferences from it.

6

Make Your Own Orthotics

For years, I wore orthotics, but when I got a different shoe (or even the same model the next year), the orthotic would no longer fit. It became expensive to replace the orthotics, so I decided to make my own. I'll explain how to do that in a moment, but first, why do so many runners need orthotics?

The arch supports in most running shoes are too low.

As you recall from Chapter 2, the typical running shoe has a lower than average arch so it can fit as many runners as possible. Over time, this lack of arch support causes the arch to either get stronger or to stretch too much, causing one of the most common of all running injuries—plantar fasciitis. This injury typically occurs with increased mileage or with old shoes that have lost what little arch support they had to start with. Poor arch support contributes to pronation, which can cause a myriad of running injuries, especially runner's knee and plantar fasciitis. This is why so many runners might benefit from orthotics.

It's easy to test for overpronation. Stand barefoot. Step forward about a foot with your right foot placing it lightly on the ground. Now shift your weight to the right foot. For many runners, the arch flattens somewhat. This, in turn, causes the ankle to rock inward—that's called pronation. As the ankle moves to the inside, the Achilles tendon also bends to the inside. As you rock forward more, the shin rolls inward. Finally, the kneecap rolls inward too.

Now, let's play that in real time. In less than an eyeblink, the following things happen—all of them bad.

a. The heel impacts the ground and then the forefoot slams down, putting three times your body weight on the plantar fascia. It can't handle the force, and the arch partially collapses. Potential injury: plantar fasciitis.

b. When the arch collapses, the ankle tilts to the inside, twisting the Achilles to the inside while it is simultaneously stressed by impact forces nearly three times your body weight. Potential injury: Achilles tendonitis.

c. The shin bone then twists violently to the inside, transferring this twisting force up to the knee. Potential injuries: Shin splints and stress fractures.

d. As the kneecap is forced inside by the twisting of the shin, it places extreme lateral forces on the Anterior and Medial Cruciate Ligaments that help the kneecap track properly. Potential injuries: Patellar chondromalacia, ACL, MCL, and meniscus tears, IT Band syndrome.

When you go for a 1-hour run, this violent explosion of energy happens 10,000 times or so.

Repeat this test, but this time with your shoes on. Ideally, when you rock your weight forward, the ankle, Achilles, shin, and kneecap should stay approximately in the same plane. If you can see significant flexing to the side, you're pronating and at higher risk for these injuries.

51

Ideally, orthotics prevent the arch from collapsing. They also might be slightly higher on the inside edge than the outside edge to ensure the ankle, shin, and knee stay in the same plane.

Running shoes try to alleviate pronation with motion control devices, but some runners still experience problems. You'll soon learn how to make your own orthotics, but there might be an even quicker fix—off-the-shelf orthotics.

42. Consider Off-The-Shelf Orthotics

If you're a large person, then motion control shoes might be right for you, but if your only problem is overpronation, an off-the-shelf orthotic might be a better solution. Here's why.

a. Motion control shoes tend to be heavier than performance shoes even after adding an off-the-shelf orthotic. A best-selling motion control shoe in my size weighs 13.2 ounces, while my shoes with homemade orthotics weigh only 9.7 ounces. That's 3.5 ounces less foot weight to lift every step, or 2 tons less shoe weight lifted in a 2-hour run. Studies show you could run a marathon about four and a half minutes faster in 3.5 ounce lighter shoes.

b. Remember, no running shoe is made to fit you. Motion control shoes tend to have higher arches, but they still might not have enough support for you. You can probably get more pronation control in a regular shoe with an off-the-shelf orthotic.

c. Most motion control shoes have a 10-12 mm heel-to-toe drop. This traditional heel drop forces you to land on your heels, which encourages pronation when the midfoot lands. Ironically, motion control shoes exacerbate the very problem they were created to solve!

I prefer a 4-mm heel-to-toe drop with a lightweight orthotic. This gives me the best of both worlds, a light responsive shoe that controls my pronation better than a motion control shoe.

43. Runners Knee and Plantar Fasciitis

Chondromalacia (runner's knee) and plantar fasciitis (sore arch or heel) are two of the most common running injuries. These injuries can be serious, taking weeks or months to heal. Motion control shoes or custom orthotics might help, but there are two less expensive options worth considering.

Off-the-shelf orthotics might provide all the support you need. An added benefit is that you might be able to switch to a lighter, more responsive running shoe. But if off-the-shelf orthotics don't resolve your problem, you can build your own orthotics. This strategy has saved me hundreds of dollars in orthotic costs. If you need orthotics, the next tip is worth the price of this book many times over.

44. Build Your Own Orthotics for 20 Cents

You can make your own orthotics for a few pennies. You'll need a pair of scissors, duct tape, and a square foot of craft's felt (available at the crafts section of discount stores). Cut the felt into a few 1½ x 2-inch rectangles. Take the existing insert out of the shoe.

Add a few of these small pieces of craft felt to the bottom of the insert in the arch area. Overlap the felt to avoid getting all the bulk in one place. Use a small strip of duct tape or athletic tape to hold the felt in place. Put the insert back in the shoe and jog a bit. If you can't feel any difference, keep adding pieces of felt until it feels like you're walking with a tennis ball under your arch. When you reach that point, it's a little too much, so remove one piece of felt. If you feel a pressure point where there is too much padding, make a mental note of where you need to make adjustments. With the shoe still on, slip your finger inside the shoe and put it on the spot where the padding must be removed.

Keep adjusting the felt by adding, moving or removing pieces as necessary. Repeat until it feels right. You want to feel support all along the arch, not just the front or the back or the outer edge. If it feels like you are running with a tennis ball under your arch, that's too much. You can use pieces of any size—just fold or trim to give support in the area you need. Most likely, you'll need 3-10 pieces on each arch, depending on how much arch support you need. Curiously, the number of pieces you need is not dependent on the height of your arch.

I have slightly below average height arches, yet I have to add extra arch support to all my shoes. Some shoe models require more additional padding than others. Also, the padding won't be the same from one model year to the next or even from your left to your right foot. My right foot needs substantially more arch support than my left and yet, it appears visually the same as the left arch. Anyway, the outside edge of the felt should stick out past the inside edge of the insert. How much it needs to stick out varies with each shoe. For me, it's typically a half inch.

On your first run, you'll probably need to make some minor adjustments. An easy way to do this is to wear a smartphone belt and carry blunt scissors, a few squares of felt, and a small roll of duct tape with you. Just stop and make adjustments during your run.

Bonus Tip: Don't immediately go out for a 10-mile run after making a major adjustment to your shoes. Test it first on a short run. It's possible to sprain the arch by providing too much support.

45. Modify Off-the-Shelf Orthotics

If homemade orthotics don't work for you, you can even modify an off-the-shelf orthotic for a custom fit. Start with a two-piece orthotic, like Superfeet inserts, and add felt between the hard-plastic bottom and foam part of the insert in the arch area.

I find that Superfeet Black plus felt work best for me in racing flats. In most performance shoes, I can just add a few pieces of felt to the existing insert.

This may sound like a lot of work, but it's faster than a trip to your doctor's office. Once you've made your own orthotics a couple of times, you can complete the entire process in less than ten minutes.

Bonus Tip: Once you make orthotics for your running shoes, you should consider making similar homemade orthotics for your casual and dress shoes as well. After all, you'll be spending more hours in those shoes than your running shoes. This is especially important if you are recovering from an injury.

46. Tilt Orthotics to Reduce Pronation

Overpronation is a major cause of running injuries, so shoe companies make two types of shoes to resolve this common problem: motion control shoes for severe overpronation and stability shoes for moderate overpronation. As you've already learned, these shoes don't always resolve the problem.

Fortunately, you can use the orthotics you made in the previous tip to also prevent overpronation.

The first step is to provide more arch support, which you can do by adding an off-the-shelf orthotic like Superfeet or building your own orthotics as described earlier. This might be enough, but you'll probably also need to tilt the foot slightly to the outside.

If you look at custom orthotics, you'll see two common characteristics. The first is that they provide more arch support than the factory insert that comes your running shoes. The second is that they often tilt the heel by raising the inside of the heel higher than the outside. This extra tilt helps reduce pronation by tilting your foot slightly to the outside upon foot strike.

You can tilt your homemade orthotic to accomplish the same thing by cutting a ¾-inch wide strip of craft's felt and running it from the back of the heel towards the arch along the inside edge of the insert. Trim the felt conform to the curve of the insert. Then, tape it in place. Put the insert back in the shoe and take a step forward as described in the "Build Your Own Orthotics" tip. If your ankle still rotates inward, remove the insert and add another strip.

Depending on your degree of pronation, you may have to add more or less felt in the heel area. On some shoes, I have to add two layers. On other shoes, I don't have to add any at all.

It's amazing how much difference this will make in the feel of the shoe.

Bonus Tip: After an MCL sprain, I had recovered to the point that I could walk without pain, but when I wore hiking boots the pain returned. Why would I be able to walk without pain in all my shoes except these? Walking mindfully, I realized I was pronating. I added one piece of craft's felt along the heel as I just described and the pain disappeared. Craft's felt is only 1mm thick, yet that tiny change in tilt of the heel fixed the MCL pain!

47. Make Orthopedic Shoes

After ten years of making my own orthotics, it occurred to me I could improve the approach by modifying the outsole of the shoe itself. My right foot pronates so badly in some shoes that adding more felt to the heel became uncomfortable, so I thought: why not tilt the entire shoe?

To do this, turn the shoe upside down. Use Shoe Goo or glue from a hot glue gun to build up the outer sole of the shoe along the inside edge of the heel. This strip should be about a ½ to 1-inch wide and about 1/4-inch thick. Start at the back of the heel and go forward 2-3 inches.

After the glue dries (24 hours), put on the shoes and try the step forward test again. It's okay to still pronate a bit, but it should be noticeably reduced. Next, run for a minute and see how it feels. If it feels like there's too much tilt, adjust it by simply running a few steps while scuffing the bottom of your shoe along the pavement. You'll grind off a little of the glue with each step. Repeat this process, reducing the thickness of the glue layer until it feels right. The great thing about the Shoe Goo method is if you mess it up, you can just peel the Shoe Goo off and start over.

Bonus tip: Once you master this approach, a more advanced method is to use a utility knife to cut off some of the outside edge of the outer sole instead of building up the inside edge. If you try this, be conservative. You can't add the outsole back after you cut it off!

I've been doing this for years, but shoe manufacturers are catching on to this idea. Several new shoe models now have more thickness on the inside of the heel higher than on the outside. This allows the shoe to tilt outward upon impact, lessening the risk of overpronation.

48. Achilles Tendinitis

Other than trauma, there are three common causes of Achilles tendonitis. Sometimes, the Achilles collar on the back of the shoe is too high, which causes it to jab into the back of the Achilles each time you plantar flex the foot (point the toe). A quick fix is just to cut off this collar. "I use a carpet knife and wire cutters to perform this modification on all my shoes," says Bill B.

However, there are two other causes of Achilles tendonitis: road camber and overpronation.

Many roads are higher in the middle than on the edges. On some roads, this difference is quite pronounced. It's called camber. Roads are built this way to allow rain to drain off quickly. If you run on the left side of the road facing traffic, this can cause problems with the right Achilles tendon because the tilt of the road forces the right foot to overpronate, pulling pressure on the Achilles.

Bonus Tip: In races or training runs, almost everyone runs on the left side of the road, but a few runners run down the middle or the far side of the road. They are probably doing that to protect a sore right Achilles tendon by avoiding the tilt of the road. If you feel a twinge on your right Achilles tendon when running on the left side of the road, try moving to the sidewalk or right side of the road if it's safe to do so.

If you routinely do track workouts, the left turns can cause problems with the left Achilles tendon. If this happens, you need more tilt in the left shoe.

49. Learn How to Use Athletic Tape

Taping has saved my competitive career. Some injuries don't respond well to orthotics. The foot, hamstring, or calf needs extra support, so I buy coaches tape by the case. I routinely tape my arches and my ankles to provide more support before every trail run, every workout in racing flats, and every race.

When someone complains of plantar fasciitis when we're running together, I'll say "Let's try taping it." Taping is a bit of an art, so it doesn't always work, but when it does, the effect is amazing. The pain disappears on the first step.

A proper taping job can alleviate plantar fasciitis, ankle injuries, and injuries to the ligaments connecting the metatarsals. Some of the athletes I coach have discovered that taping their arches provides all-day support when they're not wearing their running shoes, so it speeds the rehabilitation process.

It's almost impossible to describe how to tape an arch or ankle with only a written description. I'll post videos on this book's website to show you how to do it.

7

The Art of Stretching

Years ago, I gave my nephew, a high school senior at the time, a very expensive pocketknife as a Christmas gift. I also gave him a whetstone and carefully explained the proper technique to sharpen the knife. I then watched in amusement as he took the whetstone and did exactly what I told him *not* to do!

Stretching is a bit like that. Granted, there is a bit of an art to proper stretching, but it just doesn't seem to sink in with some runners. In fact, many runners think that proper stretching is easy. You just grab your leg and pull until it hurts and then hold it. Harder is better, so that's all there is to it, right?

Actually, if you are doing that—or if you're static stretching before running—you're doing it wrong.

Studies show that static stretching does not improve performance, prevent injuries, or reduce DOMS—delayed onset muscle soreness.

Studies show that static stretching before a workout decreases running performance!

If there are no injury prevention or performance benefits to stretching, does that mean you should avoid stretching entirely?

No, but it does mean that you may need to rethink your approach to stretching.

First, it's important to separate stretching a healthy muscle from stretching as part of a rehab routine for an injury. Let's begin by looking at stretching healthy muscles.

50. Avoid Static Stretching

Studies show that the best runners are often less flexible than their peers. Studies also show as fitness improves, flexibility decreases and running economy increases. Apparently, tighter muscles provide more elastic return energy than flexible muscles. This implies that all stretching should be avoided, but it's not that simple.

At a minimum, experts agree runners should avoid stretching cold muscles. Have you ever noticed that when you put a rubber band around something in the freezer, it breaks easily when you try to take it off? The reason is that when it is very cold, rubber becomes brittle and loses its elasticity. That's similar to what happens with a cold muscle. Since it can't stretch as far as it normally would if warmed up, there is a risk some of the weaker muscle fibers might tear.

However, if muscles aren't regularly moved through their full range of motion, they can shorten. Worse, they can shorten more on one side of the body than the other, which can lead to all sorts of injuries related to muscle imbalances. The solution is to replace static stretching with dynamic stretching.

51. Perform Dynamic Stretching Drills

Dynamic stretching is controlled stretching while moving the muscle through a range of motion. At the USATF Masters Championships, most of the top runners do some form of dynamic stretching as part of their warm-up routine.

Dynamic stretching is better than static stretching.

Dynamic drills (or stretches) put the muscles through their full range of motion. These drills include butt kicks, A skips, high knees, B skips, karaoke, scoops, leg swings, lunges, and so on followed by some easy strides at progressively faster pace. If you aren't familiar with these drills, you can see demonstrations on YouTube. I never do an interval workout or start a race without first doing these dynamic stretches. You should add these drills to your normal warm-up routine after a warm-up jog of 5-10 minutes.

52. Proper Use of Static Stretching

Although static stretching should generally be avoided prior to running or racing, there are some situations when static stretching is acceptable. This includes light stretching after a workout and the evening following a workout. Static stretching can also be done under a physical therapist's supervision when rehabilitating from an injury.

53. Stretching for Recently Injured Runners

It's not uncommon to see a runner aggressively stretching a muscle that was injured the day before. Often, they'll complain that they've had this injury for weeks and it just doesn't seem to be getting better. The problem might be they are re-tearing the same muscle by stretching it too aggressively before it can heal.

It takes about two weeks after a severe injury for scar tissue to begin to form and another three to four weeks for this scar tissue to be as strong as the surrounding muscle. Runners who attempt to stretch these injured muscles too hard or too soon increase the risk of reinjuring the muscle.

Stretching can re-tear muscle tissue if done too soon.

Thus, the best approach for a severe injury is to avoid stretching for the first two weeks to allow the scar tissue to begin to form. During this healing process, the range of motion should also be limited. How much it needs to be limited depends on the severity and location of the injury. I'll explain in the next tip.

54. Stretching for Rehab and Chronic Injuries

How soon can you start stretching after an injury? It's difficult to say because proper rehab depends on many factors. Still, we can establish some general guidelines. To illustrate this, let's look at a common running injury—a hamstring tear.

If you're a runner, chances are you've experienced a strained hamstring. It's one of the most common of all running injuries. It can also be one of the most frustrating because it tends to hang around for months. It will seem to get well and then—with a sudden twinge—it flares up again.

The reason is that these runners are re-injuring the hamstring before it can fully heal. They are not allowing sufficient time for scar tissue to form before stretching or they have attempted to return to a full range of motion too soon.

The hamstring is a big muscle so you might think it would need to be stretched pretty hard, but that's not the case.

Unless you have a really severe injury, the scar tissue itself is only in a very small strand of muscle within the hamstring. Imagine you have a dozen rubber bands attached to something. All of them are loose except for one that's tight. When you try to stretch those rubber bands, the tight one is going to break if you're not careful. That's what happens when you attempt to stretch an injured hamstring.

For hamstring injuries, you should limit the range of motion and avoid stretching for the first several days. Then you can begin to jog slowly, continuing to limit the range of motion by avoiding hills, speed-work, accelerations, and pushing off. After several days, you can begin some light stretching, going only to the beginning of tightness and then releasing after a couple of seconds.

While this approach is a good rule-of-thumb for all injuries, there are some exceptions. If your physical therapist recommends a different approach for an injury or muscle imbalance, you should follow the stretching routine your PT recommends. After all, this professional has seen your injury firsthand. However, you should always keep in mind two things. Don't stretch too hard and don't stretch a cold muscle.

55. Stretching for Older Runners

Studies show that older runners tend to lose stride length much faster than cadence. This loss of stride length is a result of two factors – decreased muscle strength and range of motion.

Decreased range of motion is a primary factor in the age-related decline in running performance.

Fortunately, strength training and dynamic stretching can reverse both of these age-related declines. Strength training for older runners is addressed later in this book, so let's look at why dynamic drills are so important for all runners.

If you don't move your muscles regularly through their full range of motion, they lose that range of motion. If you've ever worn a cast for a broken bone or a boot for a severe foot or ankle injury, you can probably remember that when you first removed the support, your muscles were very tight. It took a few weeks of rehab to regain normal range of motion.

Slow running—especially the "marathon shuffle" of many non-elite runners—doesn't move the muscles through their full range of motion.

In the marathon shuffle, the foot stays very low to the ground throughout the entire stride. The legs stay relatively straight, and the foot lands with a noticeable heel strike. This is an efficient way to run at paces slower than 7 minute/mile, but over time the muscles will shorten, especially the hamstrings, quadriceps, and hip flexors.

Here's a quick test. Stand normally. Can you lift your knee up to your chest? Can you quickly flick your heel up to your butt? If you can't do these movements, don't be discouraged. Many runners can't, but this loss of range of motion inhibits your ability to run fast. Even though the loss of range of motion is more common in older runners, it can be offset by dynamic drills, such as the ones previously described for healthy runners.

8

14 Steps to Injury Rehab

Disclaimer: I'm not a doctor. All health issues should be supervised by health or medical professionals.

A t the Huntsman World Games, I volunteered for a health study of senior athletes. When the interviewer asked what running injuries I'd had over the years, my reply was, "How much time do you have?" After I rattled off a dozen or so injuries, she remarked, "I'm amazed that you can still run!"

Over the years, I've had more running injuries than I can count. As a result, I've developed a structured approach to treating injuries that could cut the recovery time of your next injury by half. Step one might even allow a return to running the next day!

Proactive steps to treat injuries can save you weeks of training downtime.

---

56.   Pre-decide to Stop When You Feel an Injury

When you first notice a pain that might be an injury, stop running or slow down. Assess the injury. Walk a bit. Try running again. If the pain doesn't go away, abort the workout. Sometimes a tiny pain will become much worse after the endorphins of running wear off. If you are over 50, stopping is even more important because recovery from an injury takes much longer. This is not the first time this advice has appeared in this book. I'm repeating it because this seemingly simple piece of advice is so difficult for runners to follow.

I can't count how many times injured runners have told me some variation of the following. "I felt this sharp pain in my knee, so I struggled for the last six miles of my workout. Today, I can't run!" Had those runners stopped immediately, they might have been able to return to running the next day.

Stopping a working is an alien concept for runners. It requires an abrupt, complete 180° shift in thinking.

Yet even veteran runners are seemingly unable to stop when they sense an injury. The reason is that running is, by nature, uncomfortable. Runners have learned to push through this discomfort to finish their workout. In fact, finishing a marathon is considered an accomplishment even by non-runners for this very reason. Because of this mindset, stopping when runners feel an injury is extremely difficult to do.

They get so wrapped up in finishing the workout that it's difficult to shift gears to the bigger picture when injuries occur. I'll admit this used to happen to me too. Here is how I handle it now.

Long ago, I "pre-decided" that *avoiding a potential injury is far more important than finishing any workout.* With this mindset, when I feel a twinge, I have no problem aborting a workout.

Make a "pre-decision" to stop when an injury occurs. It can save weeks of rehab!

This is the first, and most important, of my 14 steps to treat injuries. When you sense a potential injury, your top priority is to avoid making it worse. Stop running immediately.

Recently, two miles into a slow recovery run with friends, I felt a twinge in my hip flexor. I asked my friends to walk with me a bit. When we returned to running a minute later, the pain returned. I told them to go on without me, and I walked two incredibly slow miles back to my car. It took me an hour, yet two days later, I returned to my normal training schedule.

If I had continued to run, chances are that the injury would have worsened, perhaps to the point of requiring several days off. On the other hand, missing one day of training is insignificant.

57. Change How You Treat Injuries

The majority of runners don't understand how to treat injuries. At best, this slows recovery. At worst, it can result in injuries worsening to the point of ending running careers.

It's important to apply the same dedication to rehab as you would to your training. It's even more important for older runners because the healing process is already going to be slower. Don't make it worse by ignoring steps that could speed the rehab process.

Everyone knows the ubiquitous mantra for injuries—RICE, or rest, ice, compression, and elevation—but they fail to understand why these are only the first stage of injury treatment.

Instead, the typical approach by young runners is IISS—ignore, ice, stretch, and strengthen! They ignore the injury at first because they've been taught that pain is something they must "run through." They don't know how to differentiate between normal discomfort and pain from an injury. As a result, an injury that could be treated with a day off becomes an injury that might take weeks to heal.

When they finally reach the point where they can't run, they ice the injury, aggressively stretch it, and go immediately into strengthening exercises. At best, this re-tears the damaged tissue, encourages more swelling, and slows healing. At worst, it tears the damaged tissue even more.

Rather than immediately attempting to stretch and strengthen damaged muscles and ligaments, it's better to apply these treatments in the proper order.

1. Prevent the injury from getting worse.

2. Restrict range of motion.

3. Provide support if needed.

4. Rehab to regain range of motion.

5. Strengthening

I routinely meet runners who lament that they can't train due to some injury. "What have you done to treat it?" I'll ask. "I've tried everything," comes the response. Yet when I ask them about the steps in this chapter, they've not done them, or they've done them wrong. With that in mind, here are the steps I take with each new injury.

Refer to this chapter after your next injury. Maybe you can find an approach you've overlooked.

---

58. Ice Immediately to Prevent Swelling

Assuming you've stopped running at the first sign of injury, the next step to prevent the injury from getting worse is icing, compression, and elevation—part of the RICE acronym—to reduce swelling. This is important because swelling restricts healing blood flow to the area.

Icing after the first 24 hours is ineffective, in my opinion, because swelling should be under control by then. If swelling returns a couple of days later, you did something wrong. You exercised or moved the injured area too much, which reinjured the area.

If swelling reoccurs, icing again will help, but you need to figure out how you reinjured the area. Then, you need to stop doing whatever you did to cause the area to swell again.

Just to be clear, my comments apply to typical running injuries, like a dinged hamstring or a rolled ankle. Severe trauma—a severely sprained ankle, for example—can result in swelling that lasts longer than 24 hours. Still, icing can be appropriate on some occasions. If your physical therapist recommends icing, then follow their instructions.

Once the swelling is under control, heat can be used to increase healing blood flow to the area.

59. Epsom Salt Hot Water Soaks

Epsom salt is an old-time remedy, but it really works. A bath is necessary for some injuries, but when it's a foot or ankle injury, I just use a clean wastepaper basket lined with a kitchen trash bag.

60. Liniment to Speed Blood Flow

I've used many liniments over the years from old school Atomic Balm to Tiger Balm to arthritis ointments. My favorite liniment is a veterinary liniment used on horses, but it has the same ingredients as the major liniments for humans.

Some runners shun liniments because they think it's a sign of weakness—implying they can't handle the pain. This is wrongheaded. Liniments will reduce pain, but that's just a beneficial side effect. The primary purpose is to warm the area, which speeds blood flow. In turn, this increases the flow of healing nutrients and carries away damaged cells.

You might already know about liniments, but are you using them? When I ask veteran runners if they are using a liniment, the answer is almost always no. The best liniment in the world won't help you if you don't use it.

61. Ibuprofen and Tart Cherry Extract

I've used ibuprofen for 20 years. Inflammation slows the healing process by slowing blood flow to the injured area. Ibuprofen reduces inflammation, speeding blood flow to the area, which in turn speeds healing. Ibuprofen should be used only in the early stages of an injury and never longer than a few days. Long-term daily use of ibuprofen has been linked to liver damage.

Bonus Tip: Some runners use ibuprofen before a workout or a marathon to reduce pain during the run. *I strongly recommend against this use.* You want to be able to feel injury pain, not mask it. Plus, it's a bad idea to use ibuprofen when you're dehydrated, which is very likely during a marathon or long training run.

Ibuprofen used to be my number one anti-inflammatory until running friends told me about tart cherry extract. It works as well as ibuprofen for me. Since there are no long-term side effects, it seems like a no-brainer to use it instead. Like many nutraceutical supplements, I have found that there is a difference in quality between brands, so I only use Life Extension brand tart cherry extract. You can buy it on Amazon.

62. Bromelain

Bromelain is a nutrient that speeds healing of bruises. You can buy it in capsule form, but I prefer to eat fresh pineapple which is rich in bromelain.

63. Aloe Vera Leaf Poultice Wraps

I've tried commercial Aloe Vera gels on injuries with no effect, but it occurred to me that perhaps the commercial product was too diluted, so I made a poultice using a real Aloe Vera leaf. It works amazingly well.

It took several attempts to figure out how to do this since Aloe Vera is very slippery. I'd put the leaf in place over the injury, and it would just slip off no matter how I tried to wrap it. It would also leave a sticky mess when it leaked through the Ace wrap. Finally, I figured out how to hold it in place.

Just before bedtime, I'd take an Aloe leaf, split it open like a hot dog bun, put it over the sore ankle, calf, knee, or Achilles and then wrap the entire area with plastic cling wrap to prevent leaks. Then, I'd wrap the whole thing with an Ace wrap. (Since Aloe is so slippery, you may need someone to hold the leaf in place while you wrap it.) The next morning, I could see an outline where the leaf was placed. The areas it touched had no redness or inflammation at all.

You'll need a mature Aloe Vera plant for this, but small plants grow fast and are available at most plant nurseries. Aloe is easy to grow. Just bring it inside when the temperature drops below freezing and don't overwater it.

In 2017, I suffered a Grade 1 MCL sprain. Typical rehab is six weeks. After no improvement the first week, I remembered Aloe wraps. In three days, the knee felt good enough to jog in a straight line. The fourth day, my knee felt so good that I skipped wrapping it. The fifth day, mild pain returned! Needless to say, I returned to the wrap and was running only three weeks after the injury—half the normal rehab time! Just to be clear, it wasn't just Aloe. I did the other steps in this chapter as well as traditional MCL rehab exercises. Still, the Aloe wraps helped.

64.   Inferential TENS Unit

An inferential TENS unit sends an electric stimulation to the injured area to speed healing. If you buy one of these devices, make sure it is an inferential TENS unit because a regular TENS unit only manages pain. They're relatively inexpensive, so every runner should have one. They're extremely portable. I'm using mine as I type this.

65.   Sleep on a Heating Pad, Electric Blanket, or LED Pad

For leg injuries, I will sometimes wrap a heating pad around the area and leave it there. At night, I will sometimes sleep with an electric blanket over my legs. It feels noticeably better in the morning. I think the added heat speeds circulation.

My friends swear by their LED light pads. I've borrowed them; they work, but they are pricey. When prices come down, I'll probably buy one.

66.   Taping

The next step in the healing process is to restrict the range of motion and provide extra support if needed. Sometimes, I'll tape an injury for a few days to provide support while the area heals and while running. Taping restricts the range of motion and provides support of the injury—the 2nd and 3rd stages of treatment. For plantar fasciitis and ankle injuries, I'll use Coaches Tape. For Achilles and calf injuries, I use the stretchy KT Tape or similar.

It's not possible to describe how to tape these injuries. There are YouTube videos, but frankly, many of the techniques don't work well for runners. I'll post my favorite taping techniques on the website for this book.

67.   Avoid Stretching at First. Add Later Gently.

In the previous chapter, you learned about the risks of static stretching, but it can still be used in the 4th stage of treatment—rehab—if you understand the physiology of healing. Let's begin by learning what happens to a torn muscle during the healing process.

In the typical soft tissue running injury, a strand of muscle tears apart. When the muscle relaxes, the ends of these torn strands come back together. Provided the muscle isn't stretched too much, scar tissue begins to form to heal these torn strands.

For the first two weeks, scar tissue is like wet tissue paper. The structure has begun to form, but the slightest pressure can tear it apart.

Here is the secret that even most experienced runners don't know about soft tissue injuries.

If you stretch too soon, you can re-tear scar tissue. The healing process must start over from Day 1. This is why some injuries take seemingly forever to heal.

To avoid re-tearing scar tissue, injured runners should avoid stretching during the first two weeks. After two weeks, if the healthy muscle tissue around the scar area is strong enough to provide support, the scar tissue might be strong enough to handle an easy workout, provided that the runner restricts the range of motion to prevent overstretching the injury. Obviously, this process can be faster or slower depending on the extent of the injury, so it's hard to be more specific.

It will take about 5-8 weeks for scar tissue to fully heal to become as strong as the muscle was before the injury. But don't despair. You can usually return to running sooner if you don't stress the weakened area. I'll explain shortly, but first, what is the proper way to stretch for injuries?

> *Common stretching mistakes include stretching too hard and stretching too soon before the scar tissue is strong enough to handle stretching.*

Avoid stretching until the pain is completely gone. You can then lightly stretch up to the point of tightness and quickly release. Avoid stretching beyond that gentle level for the next few weeks.

Stretching for injuries should only take the muscle to the first sensation of tightness and then release. Stretching beyond that point should only be done under the supervision of a physical therapist after a chronic injury. I've seen runners grimacing because they were stretching so hard. That level of stretching is counterproductive.

68. Seek State-of-the-Art Medical Advice

Some injuries simply won't respond to the treatments in this chapter. Perhaps the injury is too severe. Perhaps the pain presents as a common injury when it is actually a different injury. When this happens, it's time to see a doctor.

Many runners are leery of traditional medical advice since they'll likely hear, "Take a couple of weeks off." Most of us have already taken a couple of weeks off, which is why we finally came in to see a doctor.

A better approach is to seek assistance from doctors who specialize in running injuries or have access to state-of-the-art medical therapies. Rather than cover this information twice, you'll find tips on how to find state-of-the-art medical interventions for injuries in "Chapter 19: Advice for Masters Runners."

69. Strengthening versus Rehab

The final step in injury treatment is strengthening the healed area so the injury won't reoccur. Strengthening exercises for various injuries can be found online, so I won't go into them here.

Strengthening is widely misunderstood. If you visit running forums, you'll see many posts with the erroneous advice to immediately begin stretching and strengthening the injured area. It's a testament to the remarkable healing properties of the human body that any of these guys can still run!

Attempting to strengthen a new injury too soon can result in re-injuring weakened muscles or tendons. Aggressive static stretching the can also re-tear the injured tissue and force the healing process to start over from day one. A far better approach is to use the steps listed at the beginning of this chapter.

1. Prevent the injury from getting worse.

2. Restrict range of motion.

3. Provide support if needed.

4. Rehab to regain range of motion.

5. Strengthening

Since rapid recovery from injuries is so important for runners, let's walk through this entire process for a common running injury—a sprained calf muscle.

The first step would be to stop running immediately and ice the area as soon as possible. Range of motion should be restricted by avoiding running for a few days. Heat, liniment, and anti-inflammatories would then be used to reduce swelling and speed healing blood flow to the area. Stretching should be avoided at this stage. Once the calf heals sufficiently to run easily, the runner should limit the range of motion by avoiding hills, intervals, sprinting, and long runs. Support can be provided with KT taping and compression socks.

Rehab would then focus on recovering range of motion and sufficient strength to run normally. This should be done under the supervision of a physical therapist. Finally, and only after the injury had healed sufficiently to run normally, strengthening exercises should be started to prevent the injury from reoccurring.

Many runners start stretching and strengthening too quickly. As a result, they get reinjured.

Most runners are too impatient with injuries. They run a little; it feels okay so they tentatively run a few steps at normal running pace. When that feels okay, they just return to normal running. It continues to feel okay for a few minutes and then with no warning—ouch! The scar tissue could handle a few minutes of exercise, but not steady running. That strand of muscle has re-torn, and the healing process must start over. The problem for runners is there is often no warning. Once they feel this pain, it's too late. The scar tissue has already torn. On the other hand, stopping at the first sign of pain can prevent the new tear from getting even worse.

The question for runners becomes: how quickly can you move from one stage to the next? It depends on the nature of the injury and your propensity for healing.

A skinny high school runner with plantar fasciitis might be able to quickly move into the rehab stage and then strengthen the area sufficiently with drills to no longer need taping or orthotics. An overweight, middle aged runner might need weeks to recover from the same injury.

9

Comfort

During one of our weekly track workouts, the lack of kids in our local running scene became a topic of discussion. One of the moms remarked, "Today's kids aren't as active as our generation, so they never get outside their comfort zone with physical exercise. Running is uncomfortable for them at first because they've never felt sustained physical discomfort before." She has a point.

Americans are leading increasingly sedentary lifestyles. Running for beginners can be quite a shock to the untrained body. Although running burns more calories than almost any other sport, all that high energy means your body is doing a lot of work.

One of the secrets to enjoying running is learning how to stay reasonably comfortable at relatively high levels of exertion. The more comfortable you are when running, the more you can enjoy being with your friends or simply recapturing the joy of running itself.

Discomfort is part of running, but minimizing unnecessary discomfort makes running more fun.

70. Don't Wear Cotton

Hollywood always shows the hero jogging in a sweat-streaked cotton sweatshirt. It may look cool on the big screen, but veteran runners don't wear cotton sweatshirts when running. Even cotton t-shirts can cause problems.

Cotton is heavy. It doesn't breathe well. In other words, it doesn't move heat or moisture away from your body. That means you will get hot much quicker in the summer in a cotton t-shirt. Then you sweat—a lot. Since cotton is very absorbent, it soaks up water—or in this case, sweat—and gets even heavier.

Cotton shirts can cause chafing, nipple rash, or even bleeding when worn for long runs. If you've attended marathons in warm weather, you've probably seen runners finish with shirts soaked with blood.

A more serious concern in winter is that cotton loses about 90% of its thermal insulating ability when wet. Since cotton doesn't breathe well, a cotton sweatshirt will quickly get too hot, causing you to sweat. The sweat-soaked cotton shirt will then lose almost all its insulating ability, which can result in the runner getting dangerously chilled.

This is an even bigger problem for novices, who often go out too fast, get hot and sweat, and then have to run much slower in the latter half of their run. The lower exertion levels combined with wet clothes can quickly result in hypothermia.

Never wear cotton, especially cotton socks.

It's the same with socks. Cotton socks quickly get too hot, causing your feet to sweat, even in winter. Once the wet socks lose their thermal protection, you can easily get cold feet or even frostbite. Blisters are also more common with cotton socks since the wet socks tend to rub against the foot. So, instead of cotton, what should you be wearing?

71. Wear Technical Fabrics

Most veteran runners wear one of the many wicking fabrics—Dri Fit, Coolmax, DryLete, or whatever it's called by that company. Some runners refer to them as technical fabrics or shirts.

These fabrics wick moisture away from the skin, which helps you stay warmer on cold days. On warm days, the wicking action moves moisture to the outside of the garment where it can evaporate quicker, creating a cooling effect. By wicking moisture to the outside of the garment where it can evaporate faster, you stay dry and comfortable, while avoiding chafing and nipple rash.

Granted, some old school runners still wear cotton t-shirts. Teen runners, of course, must conform to whatever the fashion police currently dictate that kids wear, but for everyone else, technical shirts are the way to go.

Bonus Tip: Running shirts made of wicking fabrics can now be found in most big discount stores, like Walmart and Target, for $10-$20, so there is no excuse to wear cotton.

72. Run in Technical Socks

Technical socks have been the rage for several years, but the latest trend in socks has taken the lowly tube sock some of us remember from high school to an all-new level. Not only do these socks help prevent blisters, they even provide arch support.

Many veterans who try these hi-tech socks for the first time rave about them. At $12-$20 a pair, they are pricey, but you'll pay $150 or more for running shoes that last for only 300-400 miles, while the socks will last a couple of years. If for no other reason, you should buy a pair to see what all the fuss is about.

73. Have Different Socks for Different Runs/Conditions

Some runners will spend an hour trying on shoes and then grab a pair of socks on a whim because they match the shoes. Yet having the right sock is important to your running performance and comfort.

Over a 2-hour run, a 150-pound runner's feet will impact the ground about 20,000 times—each time with an impact force of nearly three times his or her body weight. What directly touches your feet for every ounce of those 8 million pounds of force? Your socks.

You've learned—or probably already knew—the importance of wearing technical socks, but are you wearing the same socks in all your shoes? In all workouts? In all weather conditions? If so, you can improve comfort and reduce the risk of injury by using different socks for different workouts.

In my quest to find the perfect sock, I have run in hundreds of socks. I discovered that for optimum comfort, you should mate socks with the shoe, the run, and the weather.

Improve comfort with different socks for different workouts and weather.

I have socks in three different lengths (below the ankle, above the ankle, and over the calf) and in different thicknesses (medium weight, lightweight, and onion skin). Each version has advantages in different running conditions.

In summer, my favorites are below the ankle, lightweight socks. They are cooler, but they still provide some cushioning and blister protection. For trail runs, I wear over the ankle socks to prevent grit and pebbles from getting into the sock. When racing, however, I prefer onion skin, below the ankle socks. They protect against blisters and add almost no additional weight, although it's not the weight of the sock itself that's a problem. It's the weight of the sweat that thicker socks will soak up during warm-up and the race itself.

Case Study: On hot days, sweat can run down your legs and accumulate in your socks. You've probably seen runners leaving track marks on the ground because their shoes were so wet. Years ago, when I ran in relatively thick socks all year round, my socks would be soaked after a long summer run. Out of curiosity, I decided to weigh them. Together, they came in at a little over 7 ounces. That's almost as much as an entire shoe!

In winter, I wear above the ankle, medium weight socks because they are warmer. On those in-between days when I'm not sure whether I should wear shorts or tights, I'll sometimes opt for over the calf socks because they're a good compromise between shorts and tights.

I've also found that compression socks help speed recovery of calf injuries, so even though compression socks are expensive, I own a few pair.

I typically buy my running socks at a major discount department store that carries several well-known brands of running socks. I'll buy a 3-pack for $8 or so. If I like the socks, I'll go back and buy a dozen pair.

Some readers will probably get a kick out of this. About 15 years ago, I walked by one of those sock vendors at a flea market. I noticed a few pair of a well-known brand of running socks mixed in with the cheap cotton socks at three pairs for only $2. I bought every pair of those running socks he had. You should have seen the look on my wife's face when I came home with 72 pairs of socks!

74.   Get Smelly Odors Out of Clothes

On running forums, one question comes up over and over. How can I get rid of the smell in my running clothes?

Sweat-soaked running apparel gets smelly fast, especially when in an enclosed laundry hamper or gym bag. Once after a hard summer run, I tossed my open gear bag onto the floor of the laundry room, planning to do the wash later. While I was gone, my cat found the bag and peed in it.

I guess he thought it smelled like a litter box! In all honesty, I can understand how he came to that conclusion. I ended up throwing the bag away.

Smelly clothes can be a real problem for some runners, especially since cold water—recommended for most technical fabrics—tends to remove less smell than hot water. Special sports detergents can eliminate the smell, but they can be expensive. Here are two inexpensive solutions, one of which you probably already have in your kitchen.

Add 1/2 cup of white vinegar to the wash. This simple tip eliminates all but the most stubborn smells. Make sure it's white vinegar. Brown apple cider vinegar can discolor clothing.

Washing with white vinegar eliminates smells.

Another product that works well for stubborn smells is OdoBan. I learned about this from a nursing home worker who said they used it to clean bedding for their elderly patients. Moms also use it to wash reusable diapers, so this stuff works.

75. How to Wash Technical Fabrics

Have you ever bought a nice technical top only to ruin it in your washing machine? I have—more than once. If just one tip in this section prevents ruining that new $80 Lulu Lemon top, you've more than justified the purchase of this book. Here's how to protect your technical apparel when washing.

• Wash running apparel in cold water only. It prevents shrinkage and color fading.

• Don't use bleach. It destroys the water repellency and wicking ability of some fabrics.

• Do not put technical fabrics in a dryer—line dry them only. A hot dryer shortens the life of the garment, weakens the elastic, reduces its wicking ability, and can sometimes shrink the garment to Barbie doll sizes. (Don't ask how I know this.) If you don't have access to line drying, dry them using the no-heat setting on your dryer.

I keep a collapsible drying rack in the laundry room for my running apparel.

• Don't wash running apparel with towels. They will pick up lint.

• Don't wash with any item with zippers open. Open zippers can snag the material.

• Put nicer garments or jog bras into a laundry delicates bag to prevent snagging the garment or the straps getting tangled with other clothing.

• As you learned earlier, 1/2 cup of white vinegar added to the wash cycle will eliminate odors.

• If you spill coffee or some other stain on your apparel, spray it with Shout and let it soak for a while before washing. Shout is amazing stuff.

Bonus Tip: For all you college guys doing your own laundry for the first time, wash dark colors with dark colors, bright colors with bright, and whites with whites.

New garments will bleed out some color on the first wash, so don't toss that new red singlet in with your white underwear. (Don't ask how I know this one either.)

76. How to Wash Shoes

In summer, running shoes can get smelly. Just touching the laces can leave your fingers feeling greasy. Some sprays promise to "kill" the odor, but they usually only mask the problem. The solution is mind-numbingly simple—wash your shoes.

Many runners are surprised to learn that shoes can be washed, but if you think about it, it makes sense. If shoes can handle running through puddles in the rain, why shouldn't they be able to withstand washing?

They can. I've washed my running shoes for years without problems, sometimes washing them twice a week in summer. The trick is to learn the proper way to wash them.

- Remove the inserts. Put the inserts in a delicates bag.
- Wash the shoes and inserts separately from other clothing. The abrasive corners can snag other clothing.
- Put each shoe in a delicates bag. Or, double knot the laces *tightly*. If you don't, they will get unlaced and wrap around the agitator of the washing machine.
- Use cold water only. This is important because hot water can weaken the glue that holds the shoe together.
- Use a liquid laundry detergent. Add 1/2 cup of white vinegar if the shoes are smelly or a small amount of OdoBan.
- Scrub off any mud before washing. You don't want to wash your shoes in dirty water.
- If there are any smudges or stains, spray them with Shout and let them sit a few minutes before washing.
- Air dry only. Do not put shoes in a dryer! The heat will melt the glue that holds the shoes together.

If you don't want to wash your shoes, another approach is to remove the inserts and stuff newspaper inside to absorb the moisture. I've heard that uncooked rice in a mesh bag will also absorb moisture in shoes.

77. Eliminate Body Odor

Some runners have problems with smelly armpits, even after they shower. I get this problem often in hot weather, but showering only removes the smell temporarily. Fortunately, there is an easy fix. The smell is caused by bacteria that isn't completely removed by normal showering. After the shower, the bacteria multiples quickly and the smell returns. An easy solution is to splash some rubbing alcohol into your hand and rub it over the armpit and surrounding area. That kills the bacteria.

Splash alcohol under arms to kill odors.

The smell goes away immediately and stays away.

Bonus Tip: If you put on the same shirt you were just wearing, the bacteria on the cloth will just transfer to your skin. Come on you college guys, put on a clean shirt!

78. Eliminate that Irritating Liner

I've saved one of the best comfort tips for last. The liners in men's running shorts can be very uncomfortable. They're either too big or too small. To get a proper fit, you have to pull the shorts' waistline up higher or push it down lower. Sometimes, liners can chafe against the upper thigh, leaving a nasty rash. Women runners report similar problems—mostly liners that bunch up.

Liners often wear out much faster than the shorts, forcing you to throw those treasured shorts away. Whether you should still be wearing those 70s-era Tricot knit, Texas-flagged, Daisy Dukes in public is another matter.

On a more serious note, in winter, a thin liner provides virtually no protection against the cold, which can result in frostbite.

Years ago, I found the solution to this problem was to simply cut out the liner and wear a brief made specifically for running. Asics makes a quality running brief—so do several other running brands. Once you switch to running briefs instead of liners under your running shorts, liner problems disappear. Even more important, once you find briefs you like, the fit is the same in all your running shorts.

Replace liners for comfort.

Some runners might scoff at the idea of removing the liner in new shorts. I say, don't knock it until you try it. A while back, I bought a pair of expensive running shorts. They looked great, but eventually, I realized when I went to my clothing drawer, I always chose another pair of running shorts.

Finally, it dawned on me that I had not removed the liner. Subconsciously, I was rejecting these shorts because they weren't as comfortable. I immediately got out my scissors, cut out the liner, and wore them with briefs instead. These seldom-used shorts quickly became a favorite.

In spring, you can often buy running shorts with cold weather compression liners at a discount. Just cut out the compression liner, and you'll have a great pair of summer running shorts. If you like compression liners, buy a pair of compression briefs and wear them under your liner-less running shorts. Once again, you get the perfect compression fit.

Warning: As you cut out the liner, don't cut out the pockets or the smaller key pocket. They're sometimes attached to the liner.

Bonus Tip: You might be wondering, "Does it have to be running briefs? No, but it's important that they are made out of wicking fabric and be comfortable while running. Boxer length performance briefs by Adidas, Puma, Under Armour, RBX, and Asics work nicely for me. Other brands probably would too, but I don't have firsthand experience with them. You'll have to experiment and find what suits you best.

10

Winter Running

When the weather is perfect, it's easy to enjoy running your favorite route, but staying comfortable in all extremes of weather is an art.

Some guys can run shirtless in subfreezing weather. If you can do that, this chapter is not for you. This chapter is for the rest of us—runners who have a hard time staying warm when the temperature drops below freezing.

Have you ever noticed that during the first rain of the season, traffic accidents increase because drivers forget how to drive on wet roads? After a few days, the spike in accidents decreases as drivers adapt to the new conditions and subconsciously remember what to do. It's the same with running.

Every fall, some runners forget how to dress on that first really cold day.

If you're unprepared for cold weather, your body compensates by going into survival mode. Blood vessels near the surface of the skin constrict, blood flow to the extremities is reduced as the body tries desperately to maintain body temperature for the core organs. Even simple tasks, such as zipping up a jacket or putting on a pair of gloves become very hard to do. Simply put, if you are freezing your butt off, you're probably not having fun.

The solution? Learn how to stay warm, but not too warm. It's harder than it sounds.

79. Dress in Layers

It's common knowledge to dress in layers, but it's still important enough to explain to novice runners. First, here's why it works so well. The base layer wicks moisture away from the skin, keeping you dry and warmer. The outer layer blocks wind to prevent heat loss from wind chill.

I have several very lightweight jackets that are just enough to keep the edge off the chill for the first couple of miles. After that, I take it off and tie the sleeves around my waist. If you hold the jacket by the sleeves in front of you and spin it like a jump rope, it will wrap itself up and fit like a belt when you tie the sleeves together.

Wear a jacket you can tie around your waist.

Bonus Tip: Don't overdress. You'll generate heat as you run. If you're comfortable before starting to run, you're probably overdressed. It's okay to be a little cold at the start; you'll warm up.

80. Warm Up *Before* You Go out

One trick to running in cold weather is to warm up before you go out. Five minutes on a treadmill or even a couple of minutes jogging in place will warm you up before you go out the door. By the time the warmth of the house fades away, you'll be running and generating your own heat.

81. Consider a Drop-off Loop

Our Saturday running group will start out with a 2-mile warm-up loop in winter. When we come back by the cars, runners can drop off jackets before going out again for the longer run.

82. Check the Weather Radar Online

Weather forecasts can be iffy, but short-term forecasts are a bit more reliable. With weather apps, you can use interactive weather radar to see approaching rain bands. Once you learn how to read the patterns, it's easy to tell whether you will be running in rain or sunshine an hour after you start your run.

83. Carry Spare Winter Gear in Your Car

Nothing ruins a winter run faster than getting really cold, especially your hands and feet. Wearing gloves might seem like a no-brainer, but check out your local running group in cold weather. There will always be at least a couple of runners who have forgotten their gloves and have their jackets pulled over their hands to keep warm. You'll even see runners shivering in shorts when they should have worn tights.

A spare gear bag can save the day when the weather suddenly changes.

Even with the best preparation, the weather can change suddenly. When that happens, you're in for a miserable hour or two. The solution is to carry a second set of gear in your car in case the weather changes before you start—tights if you are wearing shorts, long sleeve top if you're wearing short sleeves and vice versa.

More than once I've left home to meet friends for a Saturday morning run only to find the weather had changed dramatically by the time I reached the starting point. I would be okay because I brought a change of clothes, but many of my friends would not be so lucky. Nothing is worse than knowing you're going to be miserable the entire run because you didn't dress for the weather.

Bonus Tip: Keep a spare gear bag in your trunk. Stock it with apparel suitable for the season or a sudden change in the weather. In winter, I carry spare gloves, charcoal warmers, cap, headband, wind pants, top, rain jacket, and dry shoes. I usually carry a couple of pair of spare gloves. If your friends forget, give them your spare pair, and you'll be a hero.

84. Never Forget Your Shoes Again!

Have you ever driven to a workout in your sandals or casual shoes, only to discover you forgot to bring your running shoes? It's embarrassing, plus you miss the workout with your friends. Never forget your running shoes again by following this one veteran tip.

Keep a spare pair of running shoes in your spare gear bag in the trunk. You don't need to buy another pair of shoes to do this. I just put the most recently retired shoes from my normal shoe rotation into my spare gear bag.

85. The Secret to Buying Gloves

A friend asked me why her brand-new gloves didn't keep her hands warm. I slipped them on; in less than 5 seconds, I told her why. How did I know so quickly?

Simple. I put the gloves on. They felt warm, but when I put the back of my hand close to my mouth and breathed on the glove, I could feel my hot breath come right through. When you're running, the wind chill effect on your hands is significantly more than on your torso because your hands are moving back and forth. If you can easily feel your breath through the glove, it's going to be a poor glove for running.

The secret when picking out gloves is to make sure they can block your breath. If they can't block your breath, they certainly won't block the wind, so they'll be useless as running gloves.

It's also better to choose a glove that fits your fingers loosely, so they don't restrict blood flow to each finger. After all, you're not going to be picking things up when you're running. A loose-fitting glove will be fine.

86. Wear Mittens, not Gloves

I have Raynaud's Syndrome—poor circulation to the extremities—so winters can be brutal. I've searched for years to find a solution. For me, the next five tips are better than a $40 pair of high tech gloves.

The first secret is to switch to mittens. Mittens work better than gloves because they allow your fingers to help keep each other warm. Also, mittens don't fit tightly around each finger, which can restrict blood flow, causing the fingers to get cold.

Mittens are better than gloves for warmth.

Bonus Tip: Gloves or mittens that fit too tight around the wrist can cut off circulation to the fingers. If your gloves fit too tight around the wrist, cut through some of the elastic at the wrist to loosen them a bit.

87. Use Charcoal Hand Warmers

For some people, even mittens aren't enough. Charcoal hand warmers create heat by a chemical interaction when the charcoal is exposed to air. Placed inside mittens, they are the ultimate solution for extremely cold hands.

Bonus Tip: I hold the warmers in the palm of my hand inside mittens, but my friend Johnny Pryor, a personal trainer at Vanderbilt Wellness and Recreation Center, has a better idea for cyclists. "I tape the warmer to the inside of my wrist under my gloves before going on long winter bike rides. I can still use my hands, and it works great." It works because the arteries are closest to the surface on the inside of the wrist. If you keep the blood warm as it goes into the fingers, it can keep the fingers warmer.

88.   Reusing Charcoal Hand Warmers

Most winter runs will last only a couple of hours or less, but charcoal hand warmers can last for eight hours. Most runners just toss them after a run, but the warmers still have several hours of useful life left. Here's a little-known fact—charcoal warmers must get oxygen to keep working. If you put the warmers in a Ziploc™ bag and squeeze all the air out before zipping it closed, the chemical reaction stops. If you do this, you can use each warmer two or three times.

You can use charcoal hand warmers two or three times by stopping the chemical reaction.

One runner complained that charcoal warmers sometimes get too hot. Of course, if that happens, just take them off!

89.   Use Bag Balm™ or Vaseline™

When I lived in Nebraska, several runners would coat their hands and exposed surfaces of the neck and face with a light layer of Vaseline™. It did an amazing job of providing warmth. It was almost as warm as a thin glove, but it was a bit messy. Years later, I found an even better solution— Bag Balm™. It was originally created by a Vermont farmer as an ointment to keep cow udders from chafing in chilly New England winters, but it works equally well for hands and exposed skin.

Bag Balm's secret is that it contains lanolin, which leaves a wax-like coating on the skin. It's warmer than Vaseline and less messy. I often use it instead of a pair of thin gloves. It's also great for the ears, neck, cheeks, and forehead. It comes in a cube-shaped green can with a picture of a cow on it. Buy a can and show it to your running friends. Explain what it is and how to use it, but expect some good-natured kidding when you're finished. I even keep a spare can in my car in case I forget to cover my hands with it before driving to the workout.

Other products also work well to protect from wind and cold weather. "I use Vaseline Deep Moisture Creamy Formula™," says Karen Austin, a veteran marathoner, "It's like Vaseline, but it's a heavy lotion. It 's great to put on your face and hands before going out in the cold to run. It is also great for feet."

Bonus Tip: When applying to hands, be sure to cover your wrists. The arteries are closest to the surface there, and it will help keep your hands warm.

Bonus Tip: If you're driving and don't want sticky hands on the wheel, rub your palms together on a towel to remove the excess.

Bonus Tip: On those in-between days when it's not cold enough for tights, I'll apply Bag Balm to my knees and lower legs to keep them warm.

90.   My Miracle Hand Wax

After using Bag Balm for 20 years, I created something I like even better. It's as good as Bag Balm but even warmer with a waxier consistency.

My fifth secret to warmer hands is a Shea butter. I start with a chunk of organic, unrefined Shea butter—oil from the nut of an African Shea tree. It's solid at room temperature—similar to candle wax—so it can't be used by itself. I add a couple of teaspoons of coconut oil and a half teaspoon of raw Aloe pulp to 1/2 cup of Shea butter and mix it until it has the consistency of a thick paste. The coconut oil softens the mixture, and the Aloe gives it a creamy consistency. You might need to set this in full sun to get it to fully mix because coconut oil and Shea butter are both are solid at room temperature. Then, I store it in a small glass jar. If you don't like the smell of Shea butter, add a few drops of your favorite essential oil. I prefer peppermint.

Shea butter, coconut oil, and Aloe make an outstanding wind and cold weather barrier.

When cooled to room temperature, this mixture is solid, so it's easy to handle and leaves a warm, waxy feeling when applied. It's not cold when applied on a chilly day, like Bag Balm or worse, Vaseline.

If you suffer from dry skin or chapped hands, you might find this combination is far better than most hand lotions. Shea butter, coconut oil, and Aloe all have anti-inflammatory properties.

They are also common ingredients in women's' cosmetics, but cyclists might be surprised to learn they're also primary ingredients in many of the major brands of Chamois creams—pastes specifically developed to prevent saddle sores from long rides.

91. Wind Briefs

Cold weather brings a special risk for guys—frostbite of the genitals. When you think about it, it's easy to see how this could occur. Most running shorts are designed for cooling, and most cold weather tights have no extra insulation in this sensitive area. Ask any guy who has experienced this, and they'll tell you that it is definitely not fun. In fact, performance can suffer for some time afterward, if you get my drift.

Fortunately, there are several easy fixes to this problem. Some companies make wind briefs—running underwear with panels designed to block wind and provide a bit more warmth to this area. Another relatively easy solution is to wear underwear (but not cotton!) under your shorts or wear running shorts under your tights. Some guys just stick a sock in their briefs.

Bonus Tip: Twenty years ago when I lived in Omaha, veteran runners would fold a paper towel into quarters and coat one side with a thin layer of Vaseline or Bag Balm, and then put it in their shorts. It's windproof, waterproof, and feels warmer almost immediately. Of course, you might want to just tough it out, but trust me, there are places you don't want to find icicles after a run!

Bonus Tip: If you cut out the liner of your running shorts as I suggested in the previous chapter, you have a lot more options. You can wear a thicker, longer brief in winter or a very thin, moisture-wicking brief in summer.

92.   The Best Socks for Cold Weather

The first step to keeping feet warm in cold weather is to wear over-the-ankle socks. Many runners wear the same low socks in the winter as in summer, exposing their ankles. An over-the-ankle sock is a better choice because the arteries are very close to the surface at the ankles.

If your blood gets chilled before it gets to the foot, it can't keep your foot warm.

I have a friend who's a veteran marathoner and always wears no-show socks and tights that stop about 2 inches above her ankle. She's always shivering before the workout starts. I wonder why!

Of course, as I have mentioned several times, avoid cotton socks. Cotton loses all its thermal protection when wet, so as your feet sweat, cotton socks can get damp and then very cold in the latter half of your long run. Instead, wear socks made of moisture-wicking fabrics.

93.   Wear Thicker Socks and a Half Size Larger Shoe

Another trick is to wear a thicker sock in the winter. When I first tried this, it pinched my toes together, which caused Morton's Neuroma, so I switched to a half-size larger shoe in winter to accommodate the thicker sock. It works great and has the added benefit of more cushioning. You can even wear over-the-calf hiking socks if you like for extra warmth.

Bonus Tip: On the other hand, some runners might not want to buy a new pair of shoes just for winter running, so another trick is to wear two pairs of very thin socks. They have almost as much warmth as one pair of thick socks, and you can usually still wear the same shoe.

94. Consider Over-the-Calf Socks

Over-the-calf compression socks can offer some potential advantages to winter runners. They are warmer and claim to enhance circulation. I was skeptical at first, but since I have a continuing problem with cold feet, I gave them a try. They helped keep my feet warmer and helped prevent soreness the next day. Compression socks can keep your legs warm on chilly days when long tights would be too hot.

Lightweight compression socks are surprisingly cool. You can wear them in warmer weather than you might think.

I even wear compression socks on long flights or when business requires me to sit for extended periods.

95. Duct Tape the Toe Box

Older readers might remember the old retort: "That's about as funny as a screen door on a submarine?" Well, the toe boxes of most running shoes are mostly mesh, so cold air can flow right through, like water through a screen door.

Imagine wearing sandals in the winter—your feet would freeze! Yet some running shoes aren't much better. Just put your hand inside the toe box of your shoe. Then, put your mouth close to the shoe and breathe out. You'll feel the warmth of your breath. Cold air flows through that mesh just as easily, which is one reason why so many runners get numb feet in the winter.

Ignoring frostbite isn't macho—it's dumb. Frostbite can damage capillaries in the extremities and cause circulation problems as you get older. An easy solution is to wrap a layer of duct tape around the outside of the toe box of the shoe. The effect is immediately noticeable. The shoes are warmer! To keep the tape from coming loose, the tape should be wrapped all the way around the sole of the shoe, so the tape sticks to itself. This is important because otherwise, the tape will begin to peel off in the middle of your run. To keep the shoe from slipping on wet pavement, scuff it a few times on the asphalt before running to expose the adhesive on the duct tape. The thinner and more cloth-like the tape is, the better it conforms to the shape of the shoe.

A dime's worth of duct tape can cold-proof shoes.

Duct tape works, but it has two downsides. First, you look like a homeless person with all that duct tape on your shoes. You can use color-coordinated duct tape, but it's still a cosmetic drawback. I use black tape on a black shoe, so it's not quite so noticeable.

The second problem is that when you remove the duct tape, it leaves an unsightly, gummy residue. That's not a problem for me. I just leave the duct tape on the shoe all winter. By spring, the shoes are worn out anyway.

Bonus Tip: If you want to avoid gummy residue when you remove the tape, use gaffers tape. It's a duct tape that is specifically designed not to leave a residue. You can buy it on Amazon.

Bonus Tip: On really cold days, add a layer of duct tape across the entire shoe, including the laces. You can also wrap it around your ankles like a hiker's gaiter to keep the snow out of your shoe. You can rip it off when you finish.

96. Elastic Laces for Boots

Granted, you won't be running in boots, but I often wear boots in the winter, especially when I have to walk through snow to get to the indoor track. Boots can be essential in some winter climates, but my military style boots have 20 eyelets, so tightening and loosening the laces can be a hassle. I'd have to loosen each set of eyelets to get the boot on and then pull the laces tight for each set of eyelets.

After all that, the boot would sometimes be too tight or too lose, so I'd have to repeat the process.

To solve this problem, I replaced the factory laces with two sets of elastic laces. I used one set on the lower laces to snug to the boot around my foot. Then, I used a second set on the upper laces that I could open wide to make it easier to put on the boots. I can now lace up both boots in 20 seconds. Shock cord and cord locks come in colors, so it's easy to color coordinate boots and laces.

Another advantage is elastic laces help prevent lacing hot spots when you wear boots for a long time. I also use them in my hiking boots.

97. Carry a Couple of Spare Headbands

Knit caps (also called ski caps or beanies) are great in really cold weather, but if you get hot, you have only two options. You can uncover your ears, or you can take off the cap. Instead of a knit cap, consider a headband and a cap. Unless the weather is really cold, headbands are more versatile than knit caps. There are thin headbands that you can wear under your cap, thick ones that block the wind and rain, and wide ones that cover your entire forehead. You can easily carry an emergency headband in a jacket pocket, so it's there if the weather abruptly turns cold. You can also wear two headbands—one to cover your forehead and one down over nose, but not covering the nostrils, so you can breathe without fogging your sunglasses. A second headband can also double as a neck warmer when warming up.

Bonus Tip: When not in use, you can twist a headband into a figure 8 and wrap it around your wrist and over the knuckles of your hand. It keeps your hands warm and the headband out of the way.

98.   Don't Wait Until You Get Hot

If you wait until you get hot before taking something off, you'll already be sweating, which means your clothes will start losing their thermal ability. If the wind shifts, or the temperature drops, you could be in real trouble. It's easy to forget to do this, but try it, and you'll become a believer. The savvy runner unzips or removes the jacket *before* getting hot.

99.   Never Go Out with a Tailwind

In winter, always run with the wind in your face at the start so you'll have the wind at your back when you return. If you start with a tailwind, you'll get hot and sweaty going out, but when you turn around, the wind chill from the headwind can be brutal.

Years ago, that happened to me. I was running down a backcountry dirt road in Nebraska in January watching a spectacular sunset. It was below freezing, but there was no wind, so I felt fine. After the sun went down, I noticed it was getting chilly, so I turned around to head back. That's when I realized I had been running all along with a tailwind. The plummeting thermometer and the headwind had dropped the wind chill factor to 0°. I didn't even have a jacket. Within minutes, I was too numb to run. As I crab-walked sideways to avoid the wind on my chest, the reality of my situation sank in. This wasn't just uncomfortable; it was a potentially life-threatening situation.

I was too cold to run. It was a 2-hour walk home, and I had already begun to shiver uncontrollably. There were no houses nearby. My options were limited. I decided to double back to the nearest crossroad and then walk another mile to the main highway where I could flag down a car. As luck would have it, once I got to the main road I could see the lights of a convenience store. The manager gave me a cup of coffee and let me call someone to pick me up.

If you cannot avoid a tailwind at the start of a winter run, carry a light-weight windbreaker by tying the arms around your waist. It'll be there if you need it.

Bonus Tip: When running alone on long runs, carry Uber money and a cell phone. A few extra dollars can really come in handy. After running the Bay to Breakers race in San Francisco, our group went out to eat. The race was great fun, but it was one of those foggy, misty San Francisco days and I was freezing. We happened upon a garage sale, and I bought an old North Face jacket that saved the day.

100. Carry a Peanut-sized Jacket

Imagine you are miles from home on a winter run and you experience a minor injury that forces you to walk. Or, the temperature drops suddenly. In a matter of minutes, you're going to be freezing.

After my adventure in Nebraska, I carry emergency insulation with me on every winter run. A grocery bag, plastic newspaper cover, or dry-cleaning garment cover will do. Fold a couple of plastic bags until they are about the size of a peanut hull and wrap them with a rubber band. Put them in your running jacket pocket in the fall and leave them there all winter.

A dry cleaner bag makes a great spare jacket you can fold up and keep in your pocket.

You can use one of these bags to line your stocking cap if the wind chill is too much or you've sweated, and your forehead is now freezing.

You can use them to cover your gloves to provide a wind barrier or as emergency gloves if you forget to wear them. You'd be surprised at how much warmth you can get just by blocking the wind from your hands. You can also use a plastic bag to stuff inside your shirt to block the wind on your chest or use it to provide a wind barrier for your crotch.

You may laugh, but frostbite of the genitals can be serious. Frostbite pain can linger for days and can cause impotence. Now, while all the guys are running to the pantry to grab a few grocery bags, we'll move on to keeping other body parts warm.

101. Warm Only the Parts That Get Cold

The secret to staying comfortable in cold weather is to warm only the parts that get cold without overheating the rest of your body. If the rest of your body overheats, you'll sweat too much, which wets your clothes and makes you uncomfortably hot.

This is harder than it sounds because the obvious answer (or what everyone else is doing) isn't necessarily the right answer for you. Some people have severe problems with cold hands, while others can run gloveless in freezing weather. Some people get cold chests, while others get cold forearms.

Cold is also a subjective discomfort. One runner will say, "I was freezing. What a great time we had!" while another runner on the same run might say, "I was freezing. It was miserable the whole way!" If you fall in the latter category, you can stay warm without overheating by selectively choosing which areas to keep warm. Here's how you might do this depending on what part of your body gets cold.

a.   Cold feet: Duct tape the toe box.

b.   Fingers: Mittens, Bag Balm, and charcoal warmers.

c.   Chest only: Vest

d. Hands: Mittens, Bag Balm, Charcoal hand warmers

e. Forearms: On days when you're not sure if you should wear long sleeves or short, arm warmers are the way to go. You can simply roll them down without stopping if you get too warm. Some runners think they look stupid, but that's part of the fun of wearing them.

f. Head: Cap, Bag Balm, headband

g. Legs: Tights, over-the-calf socks. Do your knees get cold and sore in the winter? If so, a layer of Bag Balm on the knees can provide just enough protection to get you through the run without discomfort. It works for me.

102. Bring Dry Clothes for After-Run Socializing

If you want to go out with your friends afterward, bring a change of clothes. As you cool off after a winter run, it's easy to get chilled.

A change of clothes can help make you a lot more comfortable when meeting up with other runners for coffee or breakfast. Many of my friends change in the restroom. Most of the guys just change in the car.

A change of clothes is a good idea in summer as well, because your running gear might be soaked with sweat.

103. Make Your Own Ice Cleats

Running on snow can be beautiful. There's nothing quite like being the first person on a pristine, snow-covered trail with ice crystals hanging from the trees. Still, running on icy roads can be dangerous. There are devices you can put over your shoe to gain traction in snow and ice, but they aren't very good for stretches of dry pavement. Here is a little-known secret that can help you get traction on those icy days.

Go to a hardware store and get a bag of hexagonal sheet metal screws that are 1/4 to 3/8th inch long. Screw them into the bottom of the shoe about a 1/2 inch in from the outside edge. Three along each side of the forefoot and a couple on each side of the heel should be enough.

Use hex screws to turn running shoes into ice cleats.

There is no need to put screws in the middle of the shoes. The outside edges should provide all the traction you need. These are great for runs that will have some stretches of dry pavement because unlike devices you put over the shoe, there is no need to take them off. They will make a clicking sound on the pavement, but it's a small price to pay for safety on the ice-covered stretches. You might be tempted to put screws in the middle of the forefoot, but don't—it will make your shoes very slippery on dry pavement. It can also turn your Nike Airs into Nike Airless.

Caution: Do *not* wear these shoes on carpet or hardwood floors. They'll scratch hardwood and snag in the carpet.

Caution: Metal screws can slip on anything other than ice, snow, grass, or dirt. The screws in the heel can be especially treacherous and will slip on pavement. Use caution when walking or running until you get the hang of it.

104. Ice Rainbows in Trees

Winter—for all its miserably cold and dreary days—offers some remarkable beauty that can only be seen by those who are out in nature in the early morning, i.e., runners.

As a runner, you can see things other people never see, like ice rainbows.

If you're fortunate enough to run after a new snowfall, you can often see a circular ice rainbow in the trees in the early morning an hour or so after sunrise. If the tree has enough ice on the branches, look at the sun through the branches. An ice rainbow will form a circular ring around the sun inside the tree. The ring will be about 5-10 diameters of the sun out from the sun itself.

105. Frost Rainbows

Frost rainbows are even harder to see, but they're well worth looking for on a morning run. You'll need to look towards the sun a few minutes after sunrise across a closely mowed, level field, like a soccer field. If you look at the frost about 10 meters in front of you and directly towards the sun, you'll notice that some of the reflections off the frost are blue, red, and orange. From that point, a V-shaped, upside down rainbow will sometimes be faintly visible in the frost.

To the best of my knowledge, this phenomenon doesn't have a name, so I just call them frost rainbows. The frost rainbow is too faint to photograph, but it is nonetheless beautiful.

Once you know what to look for, you'll find yourself going out of your way to see it again and again. For some reason, it's not visible every frosty day, which only adds to the magic when you can see it.

11

Summer Running

Summer running offers its own unique joys. The days of running in the dark are over. After watching the sun come up on a Saturday morning run, you can meet your friends for coffee at an outdoor cafe and revel in the fact that you've exercised more since sunrise than most other patrons will the entire week. Often after a long run, our Saturday morning run group will lounge in the sun like cats on a window sill, swapping stories and laughing until the lunch crowd starts to show up.

Still, hot weather can be a challenge, so here are my favorite tips to make summer running more fun.

106. Wear a Cap

Wearing a cap in summer should be obvious. It keeps the sun off your head, prevents sunburn, and reduces glare. Even novice runners should know this, but I still see a lot of runners making mistakes in caps.

Not just any cap will do for running. Your cap should be mesh material to allow air to flow through. It should be a light color to reflect the sun. The underside of the visor should be black or dark blue to reduce glare.

Here's a secret not everyone knows. The cap should fit loosely on top of the head so air can flow under it. If air can't get under the cap, you lose most of the cooling evaporation effect. Of course, a running cap should be adjustable in case a wind comes up. If you already knew this, congratulations. Here are a couple more things you should know about caps.

Bonus Tip: In the summer, wet your cap before you start running. The evaporation provides a noticeable cooling effect for several minutes.

Bonus Tip: At summer track meets, it's very hard to run wearing a cap because it's just going to blow off, but you can still use a cap to keep cool. Before you race, wet the cap and put a few ice cubes under it. Wear it until just before the start. Then, ditch the cap and use one of the ice cubes to rub along the side of your neck, forehead, and forearms where the arteries are closest to the surface of the skin.

The less your body has to work to stay cool, the faster you can run.

---

107. Look for Microclimates

Running on hot, muggy days isn't fun, so look for microclimates—areas where the weather is noticeably different than locations only a few miles away. In Sacramento, California, the American River Bike Trail runs through trees alongside the river, creating a microclimate that is often several degrees cooler than the city itself. In Nashville, Tennessee, Percy Warner Park has hilly sections that are completely shaded from the sun all day long. It can be up to ten degrees cooler than downtown. Other examples of microclimates are running trails near lakes, rivers, forests, and areas that are upwind from major metropolitan areas.

Bells Bend Park is only eight miles from downtown Nashville, yet it is much cooler in the early morning because it is outside the urban heating effect of the city. I can run there at 76 degrees while my friends in the city are suffering in humid 83-degree weather.

108. Lift 2,000 Pounds Less. Wear Thin Socks.

Many runners sweat so much in summer runs that their socks are soaked with sweat. Not only can this cause blisters, thick socks can hold up to a quarter pound of sweat apiece. That's a lot of extra weight to carry around! Wear thin socks instead.

109. Have Summer and Winter Running Shoes

Why do you wear sandals in summer and boots in winter? The answer is obvious; sandals are cooler, and boots are warmer. They each fit their respective seasons. With this in mind, why should you wear the same running shoe in summer and winter?

Summer running shoes should have more mesh to allow faster evaporation of sweat. Winter running shoes should have less mesh.

In winter, I sometimes wear shoes with no mesh at all. As a result, they are noticeably warmer than my summer running shoes.

110. Wear Sleeveless Tops

A sleeveless top is cooler than a short sleeve top and better than a singlet because it protects your shoulders from sunburn, Of course, it should be made of wicking fabric and be a relatively light color.

111. Cut Your Hair Shorter in Summer

Your body loses up to 25% of body heat through the hands and head, so it makes sense to wear your hair shorter in the summer. Women can pull their hair up in a ponytail to keep it off the back of the neck to provide a little more cooling. At summer track meets, it's sometimes 90 degrees or more. Keeping my hair shorter in summer helps keep me cool before and during the race.

112. Hem Your Top

One secret to staying cool in the summer is to trim your top so it stops at the waistline of the shorts.

Most summer running tops are way too long, especially if you are short like me. When the top drops several inches below the waist of the shorts or is tucked in, air can't get under the shirt to provide a cooling effect. When the top has been cropped, air can circulate under the shirt from the bottom and can provide significantly more cooling.

You might scoff at this, but try it with an old top. You'll be amazed at how much cooler it is when running. Women might prefer to have their tops professionally hemmed, but I just cut mine off with scissors. Regardless, the cooling benefits are very noticeable.

Women might want to wear it fashionably shorter while men might want it to come a couple of inches below the waistline of the shorts, so no skin is visible when you are running.

Bonus Tip: Wear a size larger than normal, so air can easily circulate to improve evaporation. You can also experiment with different fabrics. Some breathe better than others.

113. Shave Your Legs

This tip might be a bit extreme for some men, but it is amazingly cooler in the summer. After all, hair is just a layer of fur, so getting rid of it is going to be cooler. Many male swimmers and cyclists routinely shave their legs. Not only does it help cyclists with cooling, but the absence of hair makes road rash from the inevitable falls much easier to treat. In winter, you can let the hair grow back for extra warmth.

Just try shaving your legs. If you don't like it, the hair will grow back in a couple of weeks. If your legs itch after doing this, you did it wrong. Shave with the grain instead of against it.

If you don't want to shave your legs, you can use a beard trimmer instead. It's safer and quicker.

114. Use Body Glide

In summer, sweat and skin rubbing together can cause severe chafing. One product that does a great job of preventing this is Body Glide. It looks like a stick of deodorant. Just apply it to the inner thighs and armpits to prevent an unsightly, uncomfortable rash after your summer run. Most veteran runners know about these sports glide products, but running without them can be a painful lesson for novices.

115. Carry Ice Cubes for Intervals

You can stay cooler in your summer interval workouts by carrying a couple of technical shirts in a cooler with ice cubes. Between intervals, ditch your hot, sweaty shirt and put on an iced shirt. You can also grab a couple of ice cubes and rub them on your neck, forehead, and forearms. The ice cubes will cling to the technical fabric of the shirt like Christmas ornaments. As you run, they'll fall off and go skittering across the track. You can carry an ice cube in each hand or pull one off your shirt as you run and give it to another runner. I've done many times. It always gets a laugh, but they will use that ice cube!

At hot track meets, I wear a long sleeve white compression top. To stay cool, I'll put a few ice cubes down the sleeve to the inside of my elbows. The compression holds the ice in place while it melts. I'll also put a few ice cubes under my cap. The less your body has to work to keep you cool, the faster you can run.

116. Look for Heiligenschein (Halos in the Dew)

One of the joys of running is seeing things the average person never sees. An early morning run can be almost spiritual with dew on the grass as the sun is just creeping over the horizon. It's also the only time you can see heiligenschein—a halo around your shadow. It's not exactly rare, but most people have never heard of it.

The best place to see heiligenschein is after heavy dew on closely mown grass, like a soccer field. In the first hour after sunrise when the shadows are still long, look at your shadow on the grass. You'll see a faint halo surrounding your head and sometimes the upper body. It's caused by the sunlight reflecting off thousands of tiny droplets of water on the grass. Once you know what it looks like, you can sometimes see it faintly on asphalt and other surfaces, but it is far more striking on freshly mown grass. You can even photograph it. Check out the internet for photos of heiligenschein.

12

Getting to the Workout: Car Tips

I f you're like most runners, you drive to many of your workouts. With that in mind, here are some tips I've learned over the years.

117. Keep a Spare Gear Bag in Your Trunk

Have you ever driven to meet your friends for a morning run only to discover you forgot your running shoes—or maybe even your running shorts? Maybe the weather changed suddenly, and you don't have appropriate clothing? Maybe that new running shirt has a scratchy seam that's driving you nuts by the time you get to the workout, but you don't have another shirt?

I've had all these things happen, so I now keep a spare gym bag in my trunk filled with an extra pair of shoes, running apparel, and an after-running change of clothes—sandals, shorts, and t-shirt in summer. I also include a small first aid kit.

Years ago, I rushed across town for a water running workout, only to discover I had forgotten to pack a swimsuit. I dumped everything out of my day bag and did a quick inventory—heart rate monitor, chest strap, AquaJogger belt, goggles, and flip-flops. Try to imagine a senior citizen wearing only that without laughing! Anyway, now my car bag also includes swim trunks and a towel.

A spare gear bag can salvage a lost workout.

It's especially important to carry a spare pair of running shoes in case you have a shoe-related problem.—a blister, arch pain, or hot spot on the foot from your normal shoe. (I once drove to a workout only to discover I had packed two left shoes!)

While you're at it, carry along other items that might come in handy, like a spare running cap, water bottle, an energy bar, and sunscreen. You can also carry common first aid items, like band-aids, asthma inhalers, athletic tape, ibuprofen, Swiss army knife, survival radio, alien abduction tinfoil hat—you get the idea.

118. Keep a Spare Key Hidden on Your Car

Forty years ago, I locked my keys in my car in Penwell, Texas on a Sunday night. Yes, I am an idiot.

Just for laughs, look it up on Google maps. Penwell has a post office, but no houses, at least none you can see on Google maps.

I had to break a window to get into my car. It left such a lasting impression on me that one of the first things I do when I buy a new car is make some spare keys. I give one set to my wife and put the other spare key inside a magnetic key holder and mount it someplace under the car where it won't vibrate off.

Hide a spare key under your car, so you can never get locked out!

I'd forgotten about this until a runner locked her keys in her car after one of our track workouts, so I realized it was worth mentioning in this book.

I've also duct taped a spare key under the rear tag of the car. I could just bend the tag up to get to the key. My Mini Cooper key combines the remote and the key itself, so it's too big to fit in a magnetic case. I hide the valet key instead.

If you have a combined key and remote that's too big to fit in a magnetic case, hide the valet key instead.

---

119. Hiding Car Keys While Running

Where do you hide your keys while running? Some runners put them in their key pocket, but you wouldn't want to do that with electronic keys that might get damaged by sweat. Some runners put them on top of their car tire, but that's not a good idea since it's a well-known hiding place.

Instead, here's a way to keep your keys safe and out of sight while you run. Take a rare earth magnet—neodymium—and superglue it to the "ceiling" of your rear wheel well.

Hang keys on the wheel well with a magnet.

Car keys are nonmagnetic, so put your car key on a small metallic key ring and then attach that key ring to a bigger key ring with a quick release. I use an S-Biner #4 key ring, but a simple carabiner will do. I put all my other keys on small key rings so I can easily remove one key when I need it.

When I leave my car, I attach the small key ring to the magnet in the wheel well. The wheel well is high enough that your key will be invisible to passersby. Don't leave the key attached while driving. Road debris, wind, or rain can knock it off.

120. Be Prepared for Routine Events When You Drive

Have you ever forgotten to do something but only remember it after you've gotten into your car? Do you think of things you need to do while you're driving? It happens to me all the time.

I keep small notepads and ballpoint pens in my car in case I need to add something to my grocery list or remember to do something when I get home. For example, the next tip came to me while driving to a workout.

121. Be Prepared for the Unexpected When You Drive

You never know what might happen as you're driving, so I always carry emergency gear bag in my car. This bag carries jumper cables, spare USB chargers, 100 feet of rope, bungee cords, a roll of heavy string, zip ties, two dog leashes, work gloves, screwdriver, multitool, pocket knife, flashlight, and a Dollar Store tablecloth that I can use as a drop cloth. You might be thinking, "That sounds like a lot of work!" Not really. I only do it once, and those things are always in the car if I need them.

I was meeting a friend for coffee after a workout when she pulled slowly into the parking lot. As she turned in, part of her dashboard had suddenly fallen into her lap! Apparently, someone had worked under the dash, and the screws had worked themselves loose, causing the bottom of the dash to drop off.

The car couldn't be driven as it was, so I fetched my gear bag. Using my emergency flashlight, I discovered some of the screws were missing. Using my emergency screwdriver, I removed screws for other places and reinstalled the dash. In the places where screws would no longer work, I used my emergency zip ties to put the dash back together. My emergency gear bag sufficiently impressed my friend to garner me a free cup of coffee. Win-win for everyone.

122. Be Alert When Driving

A female runner reported being followed in her car after leaving the gym late at night. She saw a stopped police car, pulled in beside it, and the mystery car kept going, but she wondered what to do if it happened again. My suggestions were as follows.

- It's probably not anyone at the gym. It's more likely someone waiting in the parking lot looking for an easy mark.

- Park under a light or area frequented by people at night.

- Put a pepper spray canister on your keychain and hold it in your hand when you walk out to your car. Be alert. Don't dally getting into your car. I'm amazed at how clueless some women are about getting into their cars at night. This is when you are most vulnerable.

- Use Google maps to find and memorize the locations of local police stations on or near your route. If you're followed, pull up to the door and blow the horn until someone comes out.

- If you're sure you're being followed, call 911 and ask for instructions.

- **Don't stop if someone bumps your car from behind.** It's a common trick to get people to get out of their cars. Instead, call 911 and drive to the nearest police station.

Bonus Tip: The world has become an increasingly dangerous place, but that shouldn't stop you from doing the things you love.

To be clear, I'm not advocating for or against the following actions, but some of my friends have handgun carry permits and have attended self-defense classes.

I was surprised to learn that women now outpace men in new handgun permit applications. Over one million women get their first handgun carry permit each year. New applications are soaring by about 1.8 million each year and are increasing at a rate of about 10% annually. Nearly 1 in 10 adults have carry permits in most states.

I recognize that many readers are strongly against handgun ownership, so before leaving, let me again be clear. I am not advocating for or against handgun ownership. My intent is to raise awareness of an option, not advocate it. If you have children, of course, you'll need to learn how to keep firearms out of their reach. You should also attend self-defense classes to learn how to use firearms safely, responsibly, and legally

123. Keep Your Valuables Safe When Running

"Smash and grab" thieves seek out areas where women are likely to leave their purses in the car, so parking lots where runners meet—parks, hiking trails, and so on—are high theft areas. These thieves are typically in and out in 30 seconds, so if you hide valuables in the trunk or in an unlikely location, chances are a thief won't have time to find them. My car doesn't have a trunk, but the back seat folds down. I put my valuables under this folded down seat.

13

Get Off the Asphalt

Trail running has enjoyed a surge of interest over the past few years, yet many runners spend virtually all their time on pavement. That's a shame when a whole new world of running is waiting.

One reason so many runners haven't discovered the beauty and spiritual aspects of trail running is that in some parts of the country, good non-asphalt running trails are hard to find. They are either nonexistent or technical single tracks (wide enough for only one runner) with roots and rocks that make them suitable only for experienced trail runners.

On the other hand, some parts of the United States are a veritable trail runners' paradise. Wisconsin has hundreds of miles of rails to trails—old railroad beds converted to wide, hard-packed limestone. Many cities have wide dirt paths beside the bike paths, so runners have their choice of pavement or dirt. Here's why trail running can help you become a better runner.

124. Trails Help Recovery

Every long-distance runner knows about the pain of running long distances on asphalt. It's as if your legs are saying, "Hey! This is as far as I want to run today!"

Trails are a great way to recover from pounding on pavement. The difference in hardness between pavement and dirt is striking. Years ago, I ran a 50k race with a 9-lap loop course that was half asphalt and half dirt road.

After 20 miles, my legs were sore, but the pain would go away when I hit the dirt road. When I got back to the pavement, the pain would return in seconds. The difference in pounding on the joints was striking. For the last three laps, I remember thinking, "Just make it to the dirt! Just make it to the dirt!"

The next day, in spite of running the longest distance I had ever raced, I was less sore than after a 16-mile run on asphalt. That made me a believer in the benefits of getting off the roads.

Plus, you see a diversity of nature on trail runs you'll never see running on highways. Compared to running on the roads, running on trails is almost a spiritual experience.

On a trail run near Sacramento, California, I suddenly came upon a huge flock of wild turkeys. They didn't fly away—they simply moved off the path as I ran by. I could almost touch them. I counted 74, but there were probably more.

On another trail run in the Sierra Nevada mountains, we had just turned around to head back when we came across footprints of a mountain lion that hadn't been there 20 minutes earlier when we passed by the first time. Carefully following the tracks, we determined it came out on the trail after we passed and was following us at a walk. But when it heard us coming back, it turned around and ran into a nearby thicket. We stood for a moment staring into the thicket wondering if the big cat was looking back at us—and how long it had been since it had last eaten!

Trail running is beautiful in all seasons. In the spring, you can literally see the forest come to life. In the fall, you can watch the leaves gradually change color, turning into a spectacular watercolor of oranges and red. In winter, when fresh snow covers the trails, you can sometimes get the ultimate gift of being the first to leave footprints in the snow. You're going where no one has gone before. Of course, trails are probably at their best in the summer, when the forest's shadows hide you from the blistering heat of the sun. It's not uncommon for forest trails to be 10 degrees cooler than the pavement only a few miles away.

Running trails strengthens your ankles and legs due to the proprioceptive forces of running on uneven terrain.

Bonus Tip: Trail running does make your legs stronger, but it's a misconception that hilly or technical running trails make you faster. Your stride and pace will be markedly different on technical trails than on roads. To get faster, you need a trail that closely approximates your typical race terrain. Still, trail running is fun, and it helps with strength and endurance.

125. How to Find Trails

In some parts of the country, decent running trails are hard to find, but if you know any ultrarunners, ask them. Since ultramarathons are done on trails, ultrarunners are more likely to know about every trail nearby because that is where they do a lot of their training runs. You may have to drive a bit, but the experience makes it worthwhile. Of course, you can also ask at local running stores and your running friends. If you are traveling to a new location, ask online at a running forum.

On a cross-country trip, I once stopped at a state welcome center and asked if there were any running trails in the state parks nearby. It turned out that a great running trail was only a couple of miles off the interstate a few miles ahead. I stopped and ran a beautiful trail that I still remember to this day.

126. Lift Your Feet and Take Soft Steps

While trails can be fun, they can also lead to more falls. Unlike roads, trails require that you watch where you put your feet. It's not as easy to break old habits as you might think. I took a veteran marathoner out for a trail run, and she fell twice in the first mile before we gave up and walked back to the road. After watching her form, I realized she had become so efficient in gliding along in marathons that her foot was barely an inch off the ground on the forward motion of her stride. While that was probably efficient for a road marathon, it was an accident waiting to happen on trails where rocks and roots could catch a foot in midstride. To become a proficient trail runner, she would have to learn to lift her foot a little higher on her forward step.

It's also a good idea to avoid damp or moss-covered rocks because they can be slippery. If you must cross wet rocks, treat them as if they were ice. Be especially careful running trails in the fall when fallen leaves can hide roots or rocks. Generally, if you take light rather than pounding steps, you'll be able to catch yourself on the next step without falling.

127. Wear Amber Sunglasses

If you run trails a lot, try wearing a pair of amber sunglasses. The tint makes the rocks and roots stand out much better than gray lenses.

128. Wear a Cap

If you wear glasses or if you wear amber sunglasses as suggested in the previous tip, glare from the sun can cause problems. When the sun is shining, you'll also need to wear a cap to keep the glare off the sunglasses. The difference is striking. If you don't like caps, consider a visor.

129. Get Discount Prescription Sunglasses

I'm rough on my prescription sunglasses, so it's nice to be able to buy them at a steep discount. My current prescription sunglasses cost only $39 shipped to my door from Zenni Optical. All you need is a prescription and a couple of measurements that are explained on their website.

130. Discover the Poison Ivy Cure

Poison ivy—like the occasional fall—comes with the territory when trail running.

Fortunately, there is a cure for poison ivy that I learned from a veteran ultrarunner 20 years ago. But before I reveal this near miracle cure, here is what you need to know about poison ivy and common treatments.

If you spend any time outdoors, eventually you or your kids are likely to run into poison ivy. The first signs are redness, itching, or non-colored bumps that are eventually followed by reddish, watery bumps that itch beyond belief. Some people are seemingly immune to it, like my wife, who weeds our garden by pulling it up with her bare hands. Others, like me, can break into a rash merely by touching a pet that has been exposed. Fortunately, there are steps you can take to prevent this common summer problem.

The best approach is to recognize poison ivy so you can avoid it entirely. Poison ivy can be either a vine that grows up the side of trees or a low-growing shrub. "Leaves of three, let it be," the old saying goes. Poison ivy has three leaves on each stalk—a center leaf on a longer stalk and two side leaves that appear exactly beside each other on the stem. These side leaves aren't attached directly to the stalk but by a short stemlet. Sometimes, but not always, the stalk and stemlets will have a slight reddish tint. Each stalk leading to a cluster of three leaves will alternate on the vine.

It's not uncommon to get poison ivy rash so bad that it requires a trip to the doctor for a steroid shot. That pain and inconvenience can usually be avoided by understanding how poison ivy works.

Poison ivy secretes an oily substance called urushiol that binds to the skin like glue. Most of the major treatments for poison ivy, like Calamine lotion and anti-itch medication, do not remove this oil from the skin They only treat the symptoms, so the itching returns. An untreated rash can last up to 4 weeks.

To cure poison ivy, remove the urushiol oil.

Although urushiol literally glues itself to the skin, it can be washed off with common, non-moisturizing soap in the first few minutes of exposure, but that isn't practical for most runners who are likely to contact poison ivy while running trails.

If you can't wash until you get home, you should wash the affected areas as soon as possible with plain non-moisturizing dishwashing detergent.

Bonus Tip: A moisturizing detergent or regular soap won't work because the purpose of the moisturizing agent is to prevent oil from being removed from the skin, so they don't remove urushiol either.

You should use cool water, because warm water will open the pores of the skin allowing the urushiol to get under the surface, making it more difficult to remove. By the way, the oozing fluids released by itching blisters do not spread poison ivy, but the oil itself can be spread by clothing that has been exposed or by your hands simply touching the affected area and then touching another part of your body. You can use a non-moisturized dishwashing liquid and a washcloth to get urushiol off your dog's fur after a run in the woods together. It's very important to wash your hands afterward.

Often, you might not notice poison ivy until the day after exposure when the rash and itching develop. When this happens, there are two non-prescription treatments that I have found to be effective—Zanfel and Tecnu Extreme Poison Ivy Scrub. Of the two, Zanfel is superior, but it doesn't work unless used exactly according to instructions. It's also pricey—nearly $40 for a 1-ounce tube that provides perhaps a dozen applications. Still, one application is a lot cheaper than a visit to the doctor and a steroid shot. I keep Tecnu and Zanfel in my medicine cabinet. Used as instructed, the itching should stop almost immediately. If it doesn't, repeat the process in a few hours. If the Tecnu doesn't work after a couple of tries, then I move on to Zanfel.

Fels Naptha soap removes urushiol if used soon enough.

Fortunately, if you use it when the rash first appears, there is a better, cheaper cure for poison ivy—Fels Naptha soap.

Fels Naptha is an old-time laundry soap that is very effective in removing stains from clothing, but it can also remove urushiol up to a couple of days after exposure. I keep a bar in the shower, and I routinely use it on arms and legs after a run in the woods. Wet the arms and legs, apply Fels Naptha, work it into a lather, and rinse. Voila—no poison ivy!

I also keep a small piece of it in my running bag. If a fellow runner is exposed, I can give it to him. Fels Naptha is hard to find in stores, but it can be ordered online for around two dollars per bar plus shipping. One bar is twice the size of a normal bar of soap and will last several months.

One final point—most people know that urushiol will stick to clothing, so it has to be washed off, but urushiol will also stick to shoes and laces. You'll need to wash them as well if you want to enjoy an itch-free summer!

131. How to Remove Ticks

Decades ago, tick bites were mostly a nuisance, but today tick-borne diseases are on the rise. Ehrlichiosis, Lyme disease, tick paralysis, and red meat allergies are becoming increasingly common. These diseases can be life-threatening. My wife nearly died from ehrlichiosis because the doctors didn't diagnose it fast enough. Its symptoms are similar to the flu, so it can easily be misdiagnosed.

Even if you don't run trails, ticks can hitch a ride inside your house on your dog and eventually get on you or your children. I check for ticks every day in the summer when I take a shower. Since I'm a cyclist, I shave my legs, which makes it easier to feel a tick on the bare skin

Even if you use tick repellents, chances are you or your children will eventually get a tick bite. The good news is ticks need to be attached for about a day to transmit disease. However, there is a reported case of Lyme disease with a tick attached for only 6 hours. Regardless, you shouldn't panic and immediately try to rip it off with your fingers as soon as you find it.

When I find a tick, I remove it using a tick twister—a miniature prybar not much longer than a matchstick. You slip the prybar between the tick's body and your skin and then slowly twirl the twister. After a couple of slow rotations, the tick releases. It's painless and much safer than using tweezers or your fingers, which can result in squeezing the tick's blood inside you or leaving the head under the skin.

I've been using the O"Tom Tick Twister for the past three years on myself and my dogs with great results. It's always left the head intact. You can buy it on Amazon. The only knock on the tick twister is that it's hard to use if you have big hands.

132. Carry Your Phone

Carrying a smartphone is a smart idea when trail running since the risk of a fall is so great. I've always hated armbands and water belts, but now you can buy smartphone belts that will stretch to accommodate your phone, car keys, earbuds, emergency cash, or whatever else you need to carry. They fit so snug you'll never know it's there unless you need it.

14

Better Heart Rate Training

I've used heart rate monitors for 20 years. While a heart rate monitor can help you become a better runner, the traditional approach to using a heart rate monitor has two major limitations. Let's look at those limitations, and then I'll explain how to overcome them.

The first problem is that to determine your training zones you first must determine your maximum heart rate (MHR). There are three ways to determine your MHR, but each of these methods has shortcomings.

The first method is to use the formula 220 minus age. At best, this only gives a ballpark number for maximum heart rate. For some runners, it's way off. For example, at age 50, my maximum heart rate was 190. The formula 220 minus age would've given me a maximum heart rate of 170. That's an error of 20 bpm—far too much to provide any meaningful training zones. Interestingly, at age 70 my max heart rate is 186, a whopping 36 bpm error if I went by the 220 minus age formula!

The formula 220 – age for max HR can be way off.

The second method requires runners to determine their maximal heart rate by doing a running test. There are multiple ways of doing this,

125

but all are extremely difficult. For example, one approach is to run 2×800m with a brief rest between intervals. The highest heart rate achieved in the second interval is your maximum heart rate. Anyone who has raced the 800m knows how hard this is to do. An easier approach is to race a 5k, pick up the pace with 800m to go and then kick in for the last 400m. This is a little easier to do and still elicits a reasonably accurate MHR, as long as the runner isn't too tired to kick at the end. If the runner is too tired to kick, then it's impossible to raise the heart rate enough to reach maximum.

The final method for runners who can afford it is to measure maximum heart rate with a treadmill test at one of the university performance labs around the country. This test involves hooking you up to an electrocardiogram and an oxygen mask and then running on a treadmill, gradually increasing the pace until you collapse. I've done this method as well. In my case, the treadmill test and the 5K test gave almost identical readings of 190 bpm.

Traditional HR training zone ranges are too wide.
Lactate threshold heart rate is a better way.

Let's assume you've done one of these approaches, so you know your maximum heart rate. In theory, you could now determine your training zones to optimize your workouts. In reality, these zones are still relatively wide and vary a lot depending on your state of fitness. They only allow you to determine your approximate training zones, which may or may not be accurate for you.

For example, the tempo zone is the most critical of all the target zones because the upper limit of the tempo zone marks the lactate threshold. If you run higher than that heart rate, the workout becomes anaerobic, and you are no longer training the aerobic system. An elite runner might be able to train at 92% of MHR, but a recreational runner might only be able to train at 80% of MHR. Again, the range is too wide to provide the optimal training effect.

Case Study: Traditional heart rate monitor zones set the upper level of the lactate threshold between 88 and 92% of MHR for highly trained runners. For me, that would be between 167 and 175 bpm. The problem with this range is that difference in pace between 167 and 175 bpm is about 40 seconds per mile for me. That's such a broad range as to be almost worthless in a tempo workout.

A better approach to heart rate training is to use the Friel method to determine lactate threshold heart rate.

Fortunately, I was able to determine my lactate threshold within two beats—169 to 171. It didn't cost anything, and it wasn't necessary to beat myself up with a near-death effort on 800m repeats or an all-out sprint at the end of a 5K. Here's how you can determine the real number you need to know—your lactate threshold heart rate—with one (relatively) easy test.

133. How to Find Lactate Threshold Heart Rate

The most important number you need to know in using a heart rate monitor is not your MHR. That number is only used to calculate training zones, which in themselves are merely approximations and can vary widely depending on your fitness level. The most important number is your lactate threshold heart rate (LTHR)—the maximum heart rate you can maintain without moving into the anaerobic zone.

The best way to determine LTHR is to use an approach developed by Joe Friel, author of *Total Heart Rate Training*, plus several other training books for runners and triathletes.

Friel's method involves warming up as you normally would prior to a hard workout and then running for 30 minutes at a pace you could hold for a 60-minute race. At the 10-minute mark of this 30-minute run, you should start your heart rate monitor. You stop it at the 30-minute mark. The average heart rate over those last 20 minutes is your lactate threshold heart rate.

As running tests go, this one is easy to accomplish, so you can do it a couple of times just to make sure the number is consistent. It's a good idea to repeat the test every couple of months. As you get more fit, your LTHR should go up a little. As you lose fitness, it goes down.

In my case, when I did this years ago with a MHR of 190, the Friel Method determined my LTHR was 169 bpm—a number that just felt right based on my racing experience at the time.

Let's assume that when you do this test, your LTHR is also 169. In your tempo runs, you would then run at a pace that allows your heart rate to gradually creep up to 169 over the first several minutes and then you would maintain that heart rate for the allocated duration of the tempo run.

Bonus Tip: On very long runs or hot days, your heart rate may creep above the LTHR towards the end of a workout. This is called heart rate creep. It's okay to let your heart rate go a couple of beats higher under these circumstances.

134. Recovery Heart Rate

A common problem with recovery runs is that many runners are competitive by nature and want to turn their recovery runs into time trials, trying to run a little faster or little further each time. This defeats the purpose of the recovery run, which is to allow the body to recover enough to do the next hard workout.

For runners who tend to run their recovery runs too fast, one way to meet your competitive urges while still maintaining a recovery effort is to use a heart rate monitor to avoid running too fast.

This raises an important question: What is your recovery training zone? Once again, the traditional method gives a wide range. However, with the Friel method, the upper level of your recovery training zone is about 30 beats lower than your LTHR. In my case, that would be 169 minus 30—an LTHR of 139.

That means I should keep my heart rate at or below 139 during recovery runs. To be on the safe side, I set my HRM to alert if my heart rate goes over 135 on a recovery run.

You can read more about Joe Friel's books and training programs at www.JoeFrielsBlog.com.

135. Lowest Heart Rate for Training Benefit

Now, you have the upper level of your recovery zone, but what is the slowest you can run and still get an aerobic benefit?

There is some controversy over this, but it appears to be about 50 beats slower than LTHR. Thus, your recovery zone should be between 30 and 50 bpm below LTHR. In my case, LTHR is currently about 159, so my recovery training zone would be between 119 and 139. Again, this feels right to me, but I usually limit my upper level to 135 on recovery days just to be on the safe side.

A heart rate monitor can help ensure that you don't run too hard on recovery days.

---

136. HRM to Determine Overtraining

Overtraining is a common problem in serious runners. If you don't give your body sufficient time to recover, you can go into a constant state of fatigue. It can take weeks or even months to recover. To ensure that you aren't overtraining, use one of the two following methods.

Run the same course at the same pace on easy days. If your heart rate is three beats faster than normal, it means that you are either sick or haven't fully recovered. You should consider taking an extra easy day before returning to your training plan.

The second method is to check your resting heart rate in bed before you get up each morning. If your heart rate is several beats higher than normal, it means that you are either sick or overtraining.

15

Competition

In the 1970s when I first started running, most people who ran were serious runners and competed often. Today, running has expanded to include millions of people who run to lose weight, maintain fitness, or to achieve something on their bucket list, like running their first marathon or running a marathon in every state.

Regardless of your reasons for running, you might eventually sign up for a race with a goal of improving your previous best time. With that in mind, let's start with some basic competition tips.

137. Race-Specific Pace Training

Regardless of the distance, if you want to become a faster runner, you need to do some training at goal race pace or faster. Experts recommend this should be at least 10% but no more than 30% of your overall mileage.

Race pace training helps your muscles adapt to the power and range of motion necessary to move at that speed. As a result, your body becomes more efficient at those speeds. That means you use less energy and less oxygen, which are major limiting factors for endurance racing.

It even works for shorter distances. Roger Pierce, a world champion 400m runner in his age group, often does workouts breaking down the

400m into two shorter distances that together total 400m. He runs those shorter distances at his goal 400m pace with only a 60-second break between reps.

For example, Roger would run 250m at goal 400m race pace, rest for 60 seconds, and then run 150m at goal race pace. For the next workout, he might run two times 200m at goal race pace with a 60-second break between the intervals.

You can do the something similar to train for your next 5k. For example, you might run six repetitions of 800m at your goal 5K pace or a little faster. To learn more about training approaches for various events, read *Daniels Running Formula, 3rd Edition* by the legendary coach Jack Daniels. It's an outstanding book.

138. Get a Coach

If your running isn't improving, consider getting a coach. Running is one of the least expensive sports there is, so if paying a few extra dollars each month can make you a better runner, why not go for it? Compared to personal trainers, who typically charge by the hour, many running coaches offer a monthly fee structure.

A coach will customize a training program geared to your training level. A coach also provides a level of accountability that is missing for a lot of recreational runners. You'll be less likely to skip a workout when you must report to your coach periodically. A coach will also see little things you might miss.

One of the first things that inspired me to become a student in the art of running was something a coach told me in 1998.

When I asked the track coach at Bethune-Cookman University in Daytona Beach if I could join his athletes for a workout, he graciously agreed. Partway through the workout, he asked why I carried my right arm at such an odd angle.

In those days, I had been training with ultrarunners who would carry their water bottles in their hands, swinging their right arm across their body to keep the water in the bottle from sloshing. I apparently developed the habit of doing it even when I wasn't carrying a water bottle. The coach gave me a simple technique to change my arm swing and sent me back out. I ran my 200m repeats a full second faster. Amazing! Granted, some of that may have been a placebo effect, but it made a believer out of me on the importance of coaching and the importance of mastering the art of running form.

In October 2002, I joined a newly formed running club coached by Jim Spivey, a 3-time Olympian. Over the next two years, 36 of our 42 members would set PRs in their chosen event. That's a strong testament to the value of a great coach.

139. Hire an Olympian as a Virtual Coach

In 2017, I jumped at the chance to attend a virtual 6-week Miler Method Boot Camp instructed by Nick Willis, a 4-time Olympian with silver in the 1500 meter run in 2008 in Beijing and bronze in 2016 in Rio de Janeiro. He is only the 8th person in the world to medal twice in the Olympic 1500 meters. The camp is co-coached by his wife Sierra, who comes from a different running background. Together, they can relate to and understand a much wider range of abilities than many elite runners turned coaches.

Although six weeks is a pretty short training period, the opportunity to train under one of the fastest milers in the world was just too good to pass up. We met as a virtual group on Facebook and shared our workout progress. It was fun, plus I got to meet runners from all over the world.

The training was a bit different than what I was accustomed to, but I followed the plan closely. After three weeks, I didn't feel I was progressing, so I discussed it with Nick and Sierra, who adjusted my upcoming workouts. At the end of the six-week virtual camp, nearly everyone ran faster. Several person bests were set in the final mile time trial. That's very impressive for only six weeks of training!

I was an exception, running the same time as before the camp. Again, I discussed my training with Nick and Sierra. They suggested a different approach for me. Although the camp was over, I followed the new plan. One month later, I ran a stunning 19 seconds faster, breaking the Tennessee state record in my age group.

I learned some valuable lessons in that camp. First, just because a training plan works for other runners doesn't mean that it will work for you. Your training plan may need to be adjusted to fit your unique strengths and weaknesses. Second, a good coach is a great investment. Although I didn't run well in my 6-week time trial, my 19-second improvement over the combined 10 weeks of training was a testament to Nick's ability to adjust workouts to get the most out of his athletes. Third, virtual camps are fun. Nick and Sierra Willis periodically run virtual boot camps on Facebook. I highly recommend them.

140. Mastering Downhill Running

Running downhill efficiently is part science and part art. On our Saturday morning runs, the entire group leaves me behind on the uphills, but I excel on downhills. Here's my secret, beginning with the science. Years ago, I saw a study that found runners used 7% more energy going up a moderate hill and 13% less energy going down the same hill. To me, that meant you should slow a little going uphill, but *speed up a lot* on the downhill.

There are two keys to fast downhills—faster cadence and changing form.

Once a downhill begins to get steep, I increase my cadence by about ten steps per minute. My arms cross a little more in front of my body, hands coming all the way to the centerline of my chest and elbows swinging a little wider from the body. This causes me to run a little more vertical than my normal forward lean. I can then heel strike instead of my normal forefoot strike, but it's not a hard heel strike. Instead, the heel touches down and then the foot quickly rolls forward. It becomes almost a floating motion.

It's very important not to feel a hard impact when running downhill. A hard impact means your foot is acting as a brake with each step. The impact also forces your quadriceps to work like shock absorbers, which tires them unnecessarily.

Regardless of how you swing your arms or how your foot initially impacts the ground, it's essential to avoid this braking force. Adjust your cadence, stride length, and pace until you get a sensation of floating. If you feel a jarring sensation, you're doing it wrong.

A key secret of fast downhill running is the ability to increase cadence and hold it for a long downhill.

To run fast downhill, you must be able to increase your cadence. However, holding a faster cadence can be very tiring unless you train for it. In the next chapter, you'll learn several competition tips I call "free speed" because just mastering the tip will make you faster without having to train harder. One of these tips is how to increase and hold a faster cadence whenever you need to do so in a race.

141. Run Faster with Downhill Shoes

As you just learned, racing on downhills can cause severe heel striking, giving you a jarring sensation with each foot strike. This puts a lot of stress on the joints and turns your quads into shock absorbers. This is why so many runners complain of sore quads after a downhill marathon. In addition to the form change I just described, one solution to faster downhills is to wear a shoe that directly addresses these forces.

Great downhill shoes either have a rocker sole or an unusually soft heel. This includes Hokas, Skechers GoRuns, and ONs. Other manufacturers make similar shoes, but these are the only ones I've personally worn.

The rocker heels of the Skechers and Hoka allow the downhill stride to land slightly in front of the heel rather than on the back of the heel. This rocker sole then creates a rolling motion onto the forefoot. It also slows the speed of the impact by few milliseconds, which lessens the pounding on the quadriceps. The ON Cloudsurfer doesn't have a rocker heel, but the cloud pods on the heel serve a similar purpose.

Rocker heel shoes help you run faster downhill.

Simply put, rocker heeled shoes will allow you to take longer strides downhill without the jarring normally associated with fast downhill running. If you race in low-heeled racing flats, you might not notice much difference, but for everyone else, the difference is significant. The steeper the hill, the more noticeable the benefit will be.

142. Want to Race Faster? Train Faster.

Studies of stride length and cadence of older runners found that cadence decreased only slightly with age. The big decrease in performance came from decreasing stride length.

In turn, decreasing stride length is caused by lack of strength and decreasing range of motion. Speedwork can help improve both of these age-related declines.

You've probably noticed that many recreational runners have only one gear. Their 5K race paces are only a little faster than their half marathon pace. These runners will complain they have no speed, but part of the reason they lack speed is they don't do any speed training. If you do all your training at 10 minutes per mile, it's difficult to race at 8 minutes per mile even over a distance as short as a 5K race.

Train slow, race slow. Add speedwork to improve race times.

Speedwork—that is, interval workouts on the track—is more specific to shorter race distances, but it can still improve your marathon times. Speedwork also increases the range of motion, so when you run faster in a race, your muscles are accustomed to this wider range of motion.

A side benefit to high-intensity exercise for older runners is that it boosts testosterone levels. Older runners should do some speedwork all year round because higher testosterone levels translate to better running performance and better quality of life for seniors.

143. Interval Workouts

To improve as a runner, at some point you need to include interval workouts. Ideally, these workouts should be on a track, but it's not necessary. When I worked out with coach Doug Butler in Melbourne, Florida, we did our interval workouts in a large parking lot where the distances had been carefully measured off.

Beginners may wonder why they need to do speedwork when they are training to run a half marathon. The short answer is if you always train slow, you will run slow.

I've met many runners who couldn't run a 5K significantly faster than their half marathon pace. When I pointed this out, they complained that the 5K was "too short" and they just didn't have the speed to race any faster. The real answer is they couldn't run faster because they had never trained to run faster.

Earlier, I mentioned that when Jim Spivey created his running club in Nashville in 2002, many of these adult runners had never done track workouts before. Our training routine involved an interval workout of varying distances each week. By our 2-year anniversary, 36 of our 42 members had set new PRs—a great testament to the benefits of interval training and great coaching.

Here's how running intervals as short as 400 meters can make you a faster runner at the marathon and half marathon.

Slow running restricts your range of motion. Muscles that move only in a narrow range tire quickly when they are asked to work outside this range of motion. Intervals train your muscles in a wider range of motion to help you run faster.

Slow running develops poor form habits that adversely affect your body's ability to run faster. The human body is a remarkable machine. If you always train slowly, it will adapt your form to run as efficiently as possible at that slow pace. Unfortunately, the form that's efficient at an 11-minute pace might not be efficient at an 8-minute pace.

If you watch the mid-packers at a half marathon or marathon, you'll see many runners moving their legs in a scissor-like fashion, barely lifting their feet off the ground. I call this the marathon shuffle. If your goal is to finish a marathon, the marathon shuffle will get you there. If you want to run faster, you might need to change your form. Intervals can help.

Intervals also train your body to utilize more oxygen. The more oxygen that gets into your muscles, the longer and harder they can work.

Intervals help maintain weight by speeding up metabolism. If you want to lose weight, adding interval workouts can help.

144. The Billat 30-30 Workout

One of my favorite workouts is the Billat 30-30, popularized by Veronique Billat, an exercise physiologist at the University of Ille in France.

The workout consists of multiple reps of 30 seconds at mile race pace followed by a 30-second jog at half that pace.

We sometimes adjust the times to allow runners to do this workout together. For example, we might run 35 seconds and jog 40 seconds, starting each new interval at the 200m marks on a track. Slower runners can reach the 200m mark just in time to start the next rep while faster runners swing wide or double back to meet the slower runners at the start of the next rep.

The advantage of starting each rep at the 200m mark is that you can see how far you are running on each fast rep. Over the weeks, you can work to increase that distance.

You can modify this workout on your own in two ways. First, adjust the time, so your recovery jog gets you to the 200m mark just in time to start the next rep. This might be 26 seconds running and 26 seconds jogging for elite runners and 40 seconds running and 40 seconds jogging for slower runners. Try to work up to at least 20-24 reps.

The second approach is just to run 30 seconds, jog 30 seconds, and keep repeating until you reach the desired number of reps. Then, see how far you ran at the end of the workout. For example, I recently ran two sets of 12x30/30, covering about 2,450m in each set. That's a little faster than a 6 minutes/mile pace during the running portion.

There are several benefits to this workout.

Billats increase the total training time at VO2 Max, a pace that is very hard to maintain for more than 5 or 6 minutes in steady-state running. Since Billats are so short, you can accumulate a total of 15 minutes or more at VO2 Max during the workout. Studies show that moderately trained runners have increased their VO2 Max by 10% in only eight weeks using the Billat 30-30.

The Billat workout trains runners to be more efficient at faster paces. This translates into faster races.

145. Blood Tests and RDAs

Monitoring your blood tests and ensuring proper nutrition is critical for racers. That's not quite as simple as it sounds.

When it comes to blood tests, normal is not a specific number, but a range, often a very wide range. It's possible to have levels significantly below the midpoint and yet still be in the normal range because they fall above the minimum value.

Runners deplete nutrients faster than nonrunners.

For example, some women have found their racing performance was impaired when their ferritin (iron) levels fell into the low end of the normal range. Many doctors assume this is okay, but coaches have amassed a significant amount of anecdotal evidence showing that female runners could reduce fatigue and return to normal levels of performance by taking an iron supplement to move closer to the midpoint of the normal range. *Caution: Iron becomes toxic quickly.* You should only supplement with iron after a blood test has shown that your iron levels that are low or low-normal.

The situation is similar for RDAs (Recommended Daily Allowances) of vitamins. RDAs are determined based on the average person. *You are not average!* You're an athlete. You're exercising for several hours each week. It's common sense that you are depleting certain nutrients and vitamins faster than a person who doesn't exercise.

Of course, vitamins and supplements can't compensate for a poor diet, so eating healthy is also important if you're a competitive runner. You'll learn more tips about nutrition and supplements in an upcoming chapter.

146. Improve Your Running Form

Look closely at runners in a local race, and you'll see a myriad of running forms. Some runners barely lift their feet off the ground. Some runners lean forward while others are vertical. Some sling their arms from side to side or rock their heads. Some have a sway in their backs. Others are hunched over. In fact, some of these running forms look downright painful, yet those runners may have run that way for years.

Now, look at the form of the world's elite runners. Their running form is quite different from us mere mortals. These elite runners flow along with graceful strides and barely seem to touch the ground. You'll notice an almost cookie cutter similarity. Sure, there are exceptions, but they stand out only because they are exceptions.

Unless you're capable of running sub-5-minute miles, you probably shouldn't try to mimic exactly how these elites run, but you can become better by running a bit more like the Kenyans.

The human body is an amazing machine. Even if your running form is inefficient and injury prone, your body will attempt to adapt over time. The problem is that as you increase mileage and speed, those form flaws can come back to bite you, creating injuries or preventing you from becoming a better runner.

The best approach is to have an experienced form coach watch you run and make on-the-spot corrections. It's also a good idea to videotape these sessions so you can see yourself and gain a better understanding of how your current running form looks.

Unfortunately, some coaches and runners believe each body adapts to the unique running gait that is most efficient for that runner. Thus, you shouldn't try to change your running form.

I disagree. The problem is that improving form is more art than science. At the individual level, form changes can sometimes be counterproductive. Rather than try to find another way, coaches say, "Don't mess with it."

Fortunately, some form flaws can easily be fixed. In the next chapter, you'll learn how some simple form drills can make you a faster runner.

16

12 Tips to Unlock "Free" Speed

With the exception of half and full marathons, most races are won or lost over the last 100 meters. In my 40 years of racing, I have never been outkicked over the last 100m of any event. I've also beaten runners who were better than me by outkicking them. My secret weapons are understanding human psychology, physiology, and the speed secrets you're about to learn in this chapter.

These speed tips don't require added fitness or major changes to your training. They're so effective they're almost like getting free speed.

147. Speed Tip #1—Understand Muscle Physiology

At the end of a race, your brain will be sending powerful messages that you can't run any faster. In fact, it will probably be screaming at you to slow down.

These messages are so strong they are almost impossible to overcome, but you will learn how to control these negative messages in this chapter. Let's start with muscle physiology.

Muscles have different types of fibers—slow twitch, fast twitch, and fibers that are in between. Your muscles don't use all these fibers all the time, so even when you are tired at the end of a race, you still have un-tapped fibers waiting to be activated. Learning how to active theses fibers will give you two massive advantages over your competition.

First, you'll know that your brain is wrong when it's telling you that you can't sprint at the end of a race. You'll know you have untapped po-tential. Armed with this knowledge and the speed tips in this chapter, you will be able to finish your next race faster. As with any technique, practice will make it better. But the brain's message is so powerful, you'll need to practice overcoming it, too. You'll learn how later in this chapter.

The second advantage to understanding untapped muscle potential is psychological.

148. Speed Tip #2—Psychology of the Kick

Learning how to kick will give you a huge psychological advantage over your competition because you know that you don't have to outrun or even race the person in front of you. All you have to do is hang on until you reach your planned point in the race to start your kick. In longer races, you can use this knowledge to relax behind another runner while letting them do the work of leading and setting the pace.

I've used this tip to beat runners faster than me by dropping back so far they thought they had the race won and they slowed down. In the Florida 10K State Championship, I was caught by a runner at the 2-mile mark. He was obviously better than me because he was talking merrily as I struggled to keep up. His incessant chatter was so irritating, I said to myself, "As God is my witness, I will beat this guy!"

By halfway, he had pulled away to a commanding 10-second lead, but I forced myself to hang on. With a half mile to go, I started my final surge. I caught him at the 6-mile mark and kicked harder because I knew if I passed him slowly he would speed up and beat me. Instead, I blew by him so fast he didn't even try. I beat him by 5 seconds and won the M60 Flor-ida State 10K Championship.

You'll learn more about the actual technique of the kick in the tip "The Art of the Kick" later in this chapter.

149. Speed Tip #3—Faster Arm Swing

"Great," you may be thinking, "I know that kicking works because I've been passed at the end of a race many times, but how can I learn to do it?" Let's start with arm drills.

Over the last 30 seconds or so of races from 800m to 10k, your legs and lungs will be burning, but your arms have just been along for the ride. Now is the time to use them. Your legs may feel dead, so start aggressively pumping your arms faster as you start your final kick. Your legs and arms are tied together in cadence, so when your arms move faster, your legs will have to follow. Once you get your cadence faster, you can reduce the effort of the arm swing.

This works with no training, but you'll be able to hold this faster arm swing longer in a race if you practice the drills during your normal workouts. Here are two ways to practice this drill.

a. On your next recovery run after you warmed up for at least a couple of miles, pick a distance—the distance between two telephone poles will do—or a set time (20 seconds is a good starting point) and simply swing your arms faster. *It's very important to shorten your stride when doing this, so you don't speed up.* Otherwise, you'll turn this into a sprint drill. Recover by running normally for a minute or so and then run this same drill 3 or 4 more times. Eventually, you'll be able to increase the distance or time at this faster cadence.

b. On your next track workout, pick a point about 70 m from the finish of an interval and significantly swing your arms faster from that point to the finish. *You'll need to shorten your stride a bit. Otherwise, this will turn into a sprint, which is not the purpose of the drill.*

Of course, in a race, you wouldn't shorten your stride, but this is just a drill to get your arms stronger to handle this workload for an increasingly longer period. When I first started this drill, I could hold the faster arm swing for about 50 meters. Now, I can hold it for at least 150 meters. At the 2017 National Senior Games 800 meters, I passed two competitors with 200m to go and beat them by over 9 seconds! This technique works.

At the end of a race, your legs are tired. Use your arms to start your kick, not your legs.

Bonus Tip: Beginners invariably speed up when they increase cadence. This gets them so tired they can only do a couple of reps. Remember, it's a drill. To prevent running too fast as you practice faster cadence, consider running on a treadmill or with another runner who maintains the original pace.

150. Speed Tip #4—One Arm Swing

Some runners swing their arms past the centerline of their body instead of back-and-forth in the direction they are running. This wasted motion is slowing these runners down. Runners who swing their arms this way also twist their torsos, because part of their arm swing is coming from the torso instead of the shoulder. This makes it almost impossible to significantly speed up the arm swing as suggested in the previous tip. To swing the arms faster, cross-body arm swingers will need to change their arm swing to a back and forth motion.

To illustrate my point, try this. First, stand with your arms straight out to each side. Bend your elbows, so your closed fists are now pointing directly ahead. Now swing your arms as fast as you can as if you are running. Since you have to twist your torso to do this, you will be slow.

146

Next stand with your arms straight down. Bend your elbows, so your closed fists are pointing forward. Now swing your arms as fast as you can as if you are running. You'll find you can swing your arms a lot faster this way.

Simply put, when your arms move faster, your legs move faster, and you run faster. This is especially true for your kick at the end of the race. For runners with severe cross body arm swing, making this form change is almost like finding free speed. Here's the drill.

Stand with your left arm slightly bent with your palm inward gently touching your pocket. The exact position of this arm is unimportant. You just want it to be in a comfortable position where you can hold it immobile while you're running. Now, run swinging only the right arm. It's almost impossible to do this while swinging the arm across the body. At first, this will be tiring because your muscles are not accustomed to moving through this range of motion. Do this for 20 seconds and then repeat the drill with the left arm. Take a break for a minute and then repeat the drill a few times. Over time, build up to several sets of one minute for each arm. You will be a little sore for the first couple of weeks as the body adapts to the new range of motion.

Bonus Tip: I've noticed that some runners, especially women, have problems at first with this drill. They move their single arm back and forth like a piston instead of letting it swing in an arc. To ensure you're doing this drill right, stand with the arms straight down with your fingers straight down Now, keeping your shoulders still, swing one arm like a pendulum forward and back. Your hand is now moving in an arc with the center at your shoulder joint. Once you're comfortable doing this, bend your elbow to roughly 90° and continue this movement. That's the single arm swing movement you want to emulate when you're doing this drill.

151. Speed Tip #5—Elbows Back

Once you've mastered the single arm swing, the next step is the elbows back drill. While running and swinging both arms, extend each elbow on the backswing as far as possible. Ideally, your elbow should come up so high that your upper arm should be almost parallel to the ground. On the forward part of the swing, make sure that your hands finish the swing relatively close to your chest instead of several inches in front of you.

As with a single arm drill, you should do this drill for 20 seconds, recover with normal arm swing for a minute or so and then repeat it 3 or 4 times. Gradually over a few weeks, you should increase the time of each repetition up to 60 seconds.

What's the purpose of this drill? The typical recreational runner runs with their hands too far in front of the body. This causes their posture to be too vertical when running. Getting the elbows further back keeps the upper arm behind the body throughout most of the arm swing. To compensate for this added weight behind the torso, runners lean very slightly forward, which means your legs generate slightly more forward force.

152. Speed Tip #6—Cadence

Decades ago, researchers found that the majority of middle distance and long distance Olympic runners took about 180 steps per minute. As a result, it's erroneously become dogma that the ideal cadence is 180 SPM (steps per minute). This is incorrect, especially for very short or tall runners. Still, if you want to become the best runner you can be, you need to work on the ability to increase cadence when necessary.

Why is this important? Some runners, especially young runners, lope along at a very slow cadence. You can even see their heads bobbing up and down because they are bouncing so much. That bouncing a) Is wasted energy, b) Increases risk of overstriding and heel striking, which can lead to increased risk of injuries, and c) Limits the ability to kick at the end of a race.

This cadence drill is relatively easy. On recovery runs just increase your cadence by about 10 to 20 steps per minute while shortening your stride, so you're not really running any faster. That's all there is to it. Do this for 20 seconds and then rest for a minute and then repeat this exercise 3 or 4 times. Gradually over a few weeks, build up to one minute.

You can track your progress by downloading a free metronome app. Run at your normal cadence and sync the metronome to beep on every left (or right) foot strike. Let's assume it's 85. Since that's every other foot strike, it's 170 SPM. Next, adjust the metronome five beats faster to 90 and sync your running cadence to the metronome. Run for 20-30 seconds and then recovery for a minute. Repeat this several times. *Be sure not to speed up when doing this drill.*

You may be wondering why I've listed faster arm swing and cadence as two separate speed secrets. Aren't they just two different ways to describe the same thing? Not quite.

The purpose of the faster arm swing is to train your arms to take over some of the workload when your legs get tired at the end of a race and to give you a finishing kick. The arm swing drill is pretty aggressive, so it is not something you're going to be able to keep up for much longer than 30 seconds. The purpose of the cadence drill is to teach your legs to become more efficient at a faster cadence and help prevent overstriding. Once you master the cadence drill, you may find you're able to hold the faster cadence for an entire 5K.

For example, when I first started the cadence drill, my cadence was 205 steps per minute in the 400m at the USATF Indoor Masters Championships. The next year, my cadence had increased to 207 steps per minute. That year, I won the silver medal by a half second. Those two extra steps might have been the difference.

Faster cadence enhances downhill running.

Faster cadence is also a benefit in downhill running. Many runners over stride when going downhill. Although overstriding is faster, it forces the quads to work as shock absorbers and worse, brakes, slowing you a little with each impact.

If you cannot comfortably maintain a faster cadence, it's hard to run faster downhill. This is one of the reasons I regularly do cadence drills. On downhills that are sufficiently steep to cause most runners to adjust their stride, I can run downhill much faster than runners of otherwise equal ability. How much faster? If I can stay within 10m of a runner going up a 100m hill, I can usually catch and pass that runner on the following 100m downhill. If you do the math, it works out to about 30 seconds per mile faster on the downhills. Given that we are otherwise very similar in ability, this is a significant advantage.

Once you've trained to maintain a faster cadence comfortably, you can glide downhill, saving your quads and passing your competition.

153. Speed Tip #7—Belly Breathing

When I converted from chest breathing to diaphragmatic breathing, I became a significantly faster runner in distances from 400m to 5K. In fact, I can literally feel the power come back into my legs when I change my breathing pattern over the last hundred meters of an 800m race. Unfortunately, it would take too long to describe the proper technique and drills. Suffice to say it's not as easy as the other drills in this book.

However, you can easily tell whether you are a chest breather or diaphragmatic breather. Stand normally and put the palm of one hand on your chest and the other on your stomach. Breathe normally. If your stomach moves and your chest remains still, then congratulations, you are a diaphragmatic breather. If your chest moves but your stomach doesn't, then you can become a faster runner by switching to diaphragmatic breathing. I suggest you look up belly breathing or diaphragmatic breathing on the Internet. There are some videos on the subject.

By the way, if your goal is just to finish the marathon or whatever, you don't need to change how you breathe. Just run and enjoy yourself!

In chest breathing, runners try to pull air into their lungs. When belly breathing, runners contract abdominal muscles and diaphragm to force air out of the lungs. The lungs then refill naturally without any conscious effort to breathe in. As you are learning this, it might help to make a Darth Vader sound when you breathe out.

Forcefully breathe out quickly. Make no effort to breathe in. Allow air to naturally flow back in slower.

At recovery paces, you might forcefully breathe out for 1 or 2 steps and then allow the air to slowly and naturally refill your lungs over the next 3 or 4 steps. If you are counting steps, it would go something like this. Hunngh! 2... 3... 4... 5... Hunngh! 2... 3... 4... 5.

When you first try diaphragmatic breathing, you're going to get out of breath quickly because your diaphragm isn't accustomed to the extra workload

Remember, this is a drill. Belly breathing is not going to help you at recovery pace. You might get a little light headed because you are getting more oxygen than you need. If this happens, just stop belly breathing until it goes away.

The purpose of belly breathing is to help you hold race pace longer. It will take a few months to transition fully to diaphragmatic breathing, but you can speed up the process by practicing belly breathing during your recovery runs.

During interval workouts, the breathing pattern gets faster. Hunngh! 2... 3... 4. Hunngh! 2... 3... 4. Breathing out forcefully on every fourth step. Once you are running at race pace, the lightheadedness will go away. To prove this for yourself, do a few intervals while breathing normally and once you are tired, focus on running tall and switch to belly breathing over the last hundred meters. I find that I'm able to finish much stronger doing this.

In my experience training other runners, it only takes a couple of sessions to see benefits to see benefits, but it will take several weeks to strengthen the diaphragm enough to maintain belly breathing for more than a few minutes. That's why you need to practice it during your recovery days as well.

Why does belly breathing work? Here are two theories.

a. Forcefully breathing out expels about twice the volume of air that breathing in does over the same timeframe. You can test this yourself. Fill your lungs with air by breathing in as fast as you can. It will take about 2 seconds. Next, fill your lungs and breathe out as quickly as possible. You'll find you can empty your lungs about twice as fast as you can fill them.

b. Belly breathing forces some of the expelled air out through your nose. Breathing out through the nose is a meditative relaxation technique. The more you can relax at a given pace, the farther you can run at that pace.

154. Speed Tip #8—Avoid Floppy Hands

Some runners carry their hands very loosely, allowing them to flop at the wrist or causing the palm of the hand to face down during the front part of the arm swing. This is not a major problem for distance runners because it probably helps them relax their shoulders and hands. But in racing, it presents a problem.

Floppy hands hinder the ability to increase cadence thus slowing you down when attempting a final kick at the end of a race.

Try this drill. Stand with your arms bent in the normal running position with your fists lightly cupped and your wrists locked. Swing your arms as fast as you can. Next, perform the same drill but allow your hands to flop back and forth. You'll discover your arms cannot swing as fast.

Bonus Tip: Avoid clenching your fists. A clinched fist creates unnecessary tension in the arms and shoulders, causing premature fatigue. Instead, cup the fingers slightly and place the thumbs on the side of your cupped forefingers. Imagine you're holding a potato chip between your thumb and forefinger and you don't want to crush it.

155. Speed Tip #9—The Art of the Kick

If you're a competitive runner, a race often comes down to the last 100m. Whether you win or lose depends on outkicking your competition over that last finishing stretch. Traditional coaching wisdom is that you just need to improve your fitness. The rationale is that as your fitness improves your ability to hold pace or increase pace over the last hundred meters will also improve. While that's true, it's also a bit one-dimensional thinking.

Learning how to hang back and kick can provide a tremendous advantage in racing. You can relax and let the guy in front do the work. Once you master the kick, you also have a psychological advantage. You know that if you hang on until the end, you can outkick your competition.

Some runners complain that they can't kick at the end of a race. It's not that they can't kick; it's that they don't know how. They've never learned and practiced the mechanics of a fast finish.

Here is the anatomy of a blazing kick.

Begin with a pronounced arm swing. At the end of a race, your legs may feel like lead, but your arms are still fresh. To start your kick, don't focus on your legs. Instead, focus on swinging your arms faster through a more pronounced range of motion. When your arms move faster, your legs must follow.

I've told this to middle school cross country runners immediately before a race and then said, "Those unrecruited muscle fibers are there just waiting for you. You just have to believe they are there and go for it. Go with your arms when I yell 'Arms!' Your legs will follow." It worked, but it would have worked better had they been practicing it for weeks.

Relax arm swing. Once you have accelerated, reduce the range of motion of the arms slightly and consciously relax them. You're still swinging your arms more than normal, but this slight relaxation will allow you to hold the kick longer. Think of it as a 99% effort, but not a 100% effort. If you try to maintain a very pronounced arm swing throughout the entire kick, your shoulders will tense up, and you will tire quicker.

Increase and hold cadence. As your arms move faster, your cadence will also increase. The faster cadence activates muscle fibers that haven't been used so far in the race. How long you can hold this increased cadence depends on whether you've practiced it. With practice, you should be able to hold your kick for 30 seconds or more. Remember, when increasing cadence, the initial focus should be on swinging the arms faster. Your arms are rested, so it's much easier to let them pull you into a faster cadence than trying to accelerate tired legs.

If you watch a high school race, the runner with the faster cadence at the finish will almost always win.

Switch from heel to forefoot strike. Heel strikers can't kick. Heel strikers can only speed up at the end of the race by overstriding or switching to a forefoot strike. If you watch slow motion videos of sprinters, you'll discover that all sprinters are forefoot strikers because they can turnover faster and deliver more power to the ground. If you are a heel striker, you should practice the ability to switch to forefoot striking at the end of a race. In fact, you are probably already doing this subconsciously.

Shift in posture and push off. Prior to kicking, your focus should be on running economically—running as fast as possible while staying as relaxed as possible. Now, your focus shifts to power. Your feet hit the ground hard and fast, the trailing knee is almost straight when you push off, the heel flicks up almost to the glutes, and your eyes no longer look 10 yards in front of you, but focus on the finish line.

Increase oxygen intake. Once you practice your kick enough to hold the faster cadence and arm swing for more than 5-10 seconds, oxygen will quickly become a limiting factor. This is where belly breathing comes in. You can get more air into your lungs and breathe deeper into your lungs where more oxygen can be absorbed quickly.

Attitude. There's also a psychological aspect to finishing a race with speed and power. You must believe you can do it. To believe it, you need to practice it.

Practice. The first few times you practice your kick, it may feel awkward because you're attempting to monitor several changes simultaneously—arm swing, cadence, foot strike, posture, and breathing. That's why these drills are so successful. They teach you how to do each part of the final kick. In the end, you'll put all these steps together.

Here's a great workout to improve your kick. Run three sets of 3 times 200m with about 90-120 seconds between reps. On the first rep, run normally for 130m and then swing your arms much faster for the last 70m. Shorten your stride, so you don't run any faster than normal. The purpose of this drill is to practice increased cadence and pronounced arm swing.

On the second rep, run normally for 130m and then concentrate on pushing off forcefully with each stride. You should slow your cadence, so you are almost to the point of bounding. Once again, you should *not* run faster. Instead, you are focusing on a very pronounced push off with each stride. If you are running faster, you are doing it wrong.

On the third rep, run normally for 130m and then swing your arms faster and push off harder for the last 70m. You'll be running much faster over the last 70m, but stay under full control, so it doesn't become an all-out sprint. After the third rep, you will be exhausted so jog an entire lap before starting the next set.

156. Speed Tip #10—Eliminate the Hunch

If you watch a local race, you'll see some runners who run hunched over. The is a common running flaw, especially among older runners. For many, it has become their normal posture.

The problem with this running form is that it restricts breathing. To see for yourself, try this. Stand with your shoulders slumped forward and your back hunched over. Try to take a deep breath. Next, stand erect with your shoulders back and your back straight. Again, take a deep breath. Notice how much more air you can take in. Running hunched over restricts your oxygen intake. With less oxygen, you tire faster and run slower.

It might take some time to correct a habit that's become normal over the years, but here's one drill to help.

Stand in a door frame or with one shoulder against a wall. Step away from the wall, bend your elbow to 90 degrees, and put your forearm on the wall with your hand facing up. Move your shoulders back and down. Take a slight step forward. You should feel some tightness in your pectoral muscles.

There are other posture drills online, but it's probably best to work with a physical therapist to correct this.

In 2017, an 80-year-old runner who was recovering from cancer surgery approached me about training. He already had nearly 50 years of running experience and routinely won his events at the state level, but he wanted me to train him for the National Senior Games Championships.

As with many 80-year-old runners, he ran and stood with a slight hunch. He was good enough to win at the state level, but at the national level, this one form flaw might cost him a medal.

My challenge was to come up with a training program that would allow him to gradually improve the running form that served him so successfully for the past half-century.

Practicing the drills in this chapter, Ted Wilson stood tall at the national championships, winning bronze in the 200 and 1500 meters and silver in the 400 meters with a stunning time of 1:27.0—the 17th fastest time in the world in 2017 at age 80!

157. Speed Tip #11—Train the Brain to Endure the Pain

A while back, a successful D1 runner and now coach was remarking how other runners were faster in training, but how I would beat them in a race. I responded, "John, the reason you and I are faster in races is that we can endure more pain than they can."

Competitive runners typically improve as the season goes on. Conventional wisdom is that this performance increase is due to increased fitness. Yes, that's part of it, but racing also trains the brain to endure more pain.

The first race of the season can be such a shock to the system that the brain's messages to slow down are too powerful to overcome. By the third race of the season, runners have adapted to the shock of racing and can control these limiting messages.

In *Brain Training for Running*, Matt Fitzgerald explains how he will enter a race a few weeks before his major event with the objective of enduring as much pain as possible, rather than focusing exclusively on time. This prepares him to control the pain during the major race.

Coaches sometimes have runners do a time trial before a major race. The time trial gives runners an idea of their current fitness, but it has an even more important effect. It trains runners to endure the pain they'll experience in the race.

In the final weeks before racing the 800 meters, I'll do some brutal workouts. Often, I miss my time goals, but those workouts were still successful because they *trained my brain to endure the pain* of the upcoming race.

158. Speed Tip #12—Practice on Recovery Runs

One way to make your recovery runs more fun is to break them into sections and work on these speed tips. For example, on a 4-mile recovery run, you might run the first couple of miles normally to warm up and then do a series of low key drills over the remaining 2 miles. You might practice increasing cadence for 20 seconds and then run normally for a minute to recover. Repeat this drill a few times. Then, practice single arm swing for 20 seconds, again recovering for a minute between reps. You can use the same approach to practice breathing, forefoot strike, and pushing off.

Practice form drills on recovery runs to race faster.

As you practice your running form drills, the miles melt away. It makes slow recovery runs more fun.

17

Advice for Beginners

Running is one of the best lifelong hobbies. It keeps you healthy, reduces stress, slows aging, and controls weight. It's also inexpensive compared to other sports. You don't need golf clubs, fishing lures, racquets, gym memberships, or team gear. You don't need to reserve tee times or pay to play. You don't need to own a boat. You just need good running shoes.

Not surprisingly, more middle-aged adults are increasingly attracted to running for these reasons. According to the National Sporting Goods Association, the number of occasional runners—defined as running more than 25 times a year—is increasing at a rate of nearly one million runners a year.

At first glance, this appears to be positive news, but the same survey found the number of frequent runners—defined as running more than 110 times a year or about twice a week—is increasing at less than half that rate. Even more troubling, the total number of runners is barely increasing at all.

That means many of these occasional runners are dropping out of the sport. Why? There are two primary reasons. The first is injuries. Surveys show over half of runners training for their first marathon drop out due to injuries prior to the race. The second reason is that running just isn't fun for them.

The mission of this book is to help these runners avoid injuries, recover faster if they are injured, and make running more fun so it can become a lifelong healthy habit.

159. Be Proactive about Shoes

Beginners should definitely buy their shoes from an experienced salesperson in a specialty running store. Don't go to a place where the sales staff aren't runners. That said, don't just passively accept the first pair of shoes you try on. Try on several pairs. Be assertive. Describe your situation. Ask for a gait analysis. Tell the salesperson that if the shoes cause you problems, you will be returning them, but if you get a great fit, you'll refer others in your running group to them.

Some runners hesitate to return shoes, but here's the secret you need to know about retail sales. Running stores don't make much money when they sell you a pair of shoes. They make their money by repeat customers. Experienced salespeople want you as a repeat customer and will go out of their way to make sure you get a shoe that fits as comfortably as possible.

Of course, Chapter 2 covered shoes in detail, so be sure to review that chapter before buying your new shoes. By the way, if the advice you get from a salesperson differs from the advice in Chapter 2 and you are confident the salesperson is experienced enough to know what they are talking about, defer to their advice instead of mine. Remember, the salesperson has seen you and talked with you about your specific needs, and I have not.

Bonus Tip: Remember to take the socks you'll be wearing when running when you try on shoes. Anticipate that your running shoe will be a half to a full size larger than your normal shoe.

160. Join a Group

It is much more fun to run with a group. You'll make new friends, and it helps the time go by. Many of my friends have run with the same people for over 20 years. Groups usually have an informal training schedule and may even provide limited coaching. Equally important, running with a group provides accountability and motivation to show up on those dreary days when you don't want to run.

If you're introverted, don't worry. Running triggers endorphins that will have everyone chatting like old friends, especially if you meet afterward for coffee or a meal.

161. Get a Coach

A coach isn't just for elite runners. A coach will provide a training plan to reach your goal, help you evaluate your progress, and adjust your training plan as needed. Even veterans will tell you it's difficult to be objective about your training. We tend to get so wrapped up in staying on schedule or finishing a specific workout that we lose sight of the big picture. A coach can provide an objective, experienced evaluation of your training.

Of course, a coach also provides accountability and motivation. It's harder to skip a workout when you know that you have to report it to your coach.

Bonus Tip: Most coaches don't provide form training. You might want to ask about this in advance. It's not a deal-killer because very few coaches do it anyway, but it does mean you should read this book very carefully to ensure your running form is not increasing your risk of future injuries.

162. Dynamic Stretching before Running

A common mistake of both beginners and veterans is not warming up properly before running.

Running, especially slow running, moves the muscles through a very narrow range of motion. Over time, this restricted range of motion leads to muscle imbalances and increases the risk of injury.

The solution is to move those muscles through an extended range of motion. Many runners attempt to do this with static stretches, but this is not the best approach. Studies show that static stretching can be counterproductive to running performance and can even make existing injuries worse.

For a refresher on what happens when runners stretch the wrong way, beginners should re-read Chapter 7 "The Art of Stretching." Briefly, you should avoid static stretching of cold muscles.

Static stretching can tear cold muscle tissue.

A better approach is to warm up first and then do a routine of dynamic stretches. Before a workout, I'll jog for 10 minutes or so to get the muscles warm and then do several dynamic stretching drills. These drills include butt kicks, high knees, scoops, side skips, karaoke, A skips, lunges, adductor stretches, leg swings, and strides. It's much easier to learn how to do these dynamic stretches by watching a video. You can find videos online.

163. Marathons—Respect the Distance

Many novices join the running movement with a goal of eventually running a marathon. While this might be a good bucket list goal and a great way to stay motivated at first, it can be detrimental to making running a lifelong sport. Novices tend to make four common mistakes when running a marathon. They'll be covered in the next four tips, beginning with attempting to do too much too soon.

I've seen training plans that take runners from a long run of 5 miles to running a marathon in 18 weeks. Yes, it's possible because tens of thousands of runners have done it, but in my opinion, beginners should take a more conservative approach.

To me, short marathon training programs set up runners for failure Over half of first-time marathoners get injured badly enough to prevent running the event. Second, running should be fun. It's not fun to increase mileage from a very low baseline to running 26.2 miles in only 18 weeks.

These runners might survive the training to finish the marathon, but the experience is likely to be so uncomfortable that they won't enjoy it. As a result, many of them drop out of running after they check the marathon off their bucket list. That's sad since running can be such a healthy, lifetime exercise.

A better approach for novice marathoners is to train at least six months to run a half marathon and then continue to run half marathons until they can run it in 2:15 or less. Once novices reach this level, they could train to run a marathon in about nine months.

Marathons are not for everyone. You can be a runner without running marathons.

By the way, not everyone is genetically gifted to run a marathon, just as not everyone can become a great sprinter. The marathon does have a certain mystique and it's nice to be able to say "yes" when non-runners ask if you've run a marathon. But the marathon might not be the best distance for you. Run a marathon to check it off your bucket list if you must, but don't rush the training and don't let the marathon define you as a runner. Don't let peer pressure coerce you into training for a marathon before you're ready. Running should be fun.

164. Take Walk Breaks

A typical novice mistake in their first marathon is to run as far as possible and then walk the last few miles. A faster and less painful approach is to build walk breaks into your training. Walk breaks were popularized by Jeff Galloway, the 1972 Olympic marathon gold medalist. Using this approach, sometimes referred to as Gallowalking, thousands of beginners have built up enough endurance to run a marathon.

A typical approach might be to run for 7 minutes and then take a 1-minute walk break. Building walk breaks into your run has several advantages.

a.   It allows runners of different abilities to train together.

b.   Beginners can run farther with less risk of injury.

c.   Your legs will feel less sore the next day.

d.   The brief recovery keeps your form from deteriorating due to fatigue—a leading cause of injury.

Recently, I went for a run with several friends who were faster than me. When I could no longer maintain their pace, I took a walk break and then resumed running on my own, taking a brief walk break every mile. This ensured that my form didn't break down, which I've learned from experience is a prescription for injury. Not only did I maintain my form, but my legs were also less tired afterward.

Whether walk breaks make you faster is a matter of ferocious debate on running forums, but it definitely helps some runners. In fact, some of my training partners have qualified for the prestigious Boston marathon by taking walk breaks, passing dozens of runners over the last few miles of the race.

I haven't raced a marathon for many years, but I'm a believer in the Galloway method. As a test, I ran a 4-mile tempo, getting my heart rate up to my personal target of 169 beats per minute and holding it there for the entire workout. Later, I did the same 4-mile tempo taking 1-minute walk breaks every 5 minutes. In spite of 4 minutes walking, my overall time was only 30 seconds slower. Even more impressive, my average heart rate was four beats per minute lower with walk breaks. This is a huge difference and indicates that my body had to do less work on the run with walk breaks. I also felt less tired the next day.

If you're training for your first marathon, you should consider using walk breaks in your training and in the marathon itself.

As a beginner, you may be <u>faster</u> with walk breaks!

As a beginner, it's likely you will be faster with walk breaks because you will slow down less over the last few miles. It's not uncommon to see runners stay on their goal marathon pace for 20 miles only to slow to a survival shuffle for the last few miles.

165. Attempting to Stay on Schedule at All Costs

For beginners and many veterans, the mantra is "Stay on the training schedule. Work through the pain! Finish the marathon at all costs."

This is bad advice. The marathon is a fickle race—more so than any other distance. A few extra degrees of heat can have a devastating effect on your performance. A minor injury can get far worse over the miles. I know several runners who have been seriously or permanently injured running marathons when they should have stopped.

Elite marathoners routinely DNF when they experience a serious problem. Listen to your body and follow their lead. Remember, there will always be another marathon; you only have one body.

166. Avoid Hot Weather Marathons

The fourth common marathon mistake is running a marathon in hot weather. Yet runners who have booked hotels, airfare and paid nonrefundable entry fees are ill-disposed to drop out of the race. Some are stubborn, but others are afraid they will be seen as quitters.

Because the marathon works the body so hard for so long, even moderate temperatures—that is, a temperature above 70 degrees—can result in heat stroke, heat exhaustion, dehydration, or hyponatremia. It's not just the heat. Moderately high humidity and lack of cloud cover can combine to adversely affect the body's ability to cool itself.

Heat stroke can cause permanent damage to the heart, liver, kidneys, or brain. An even more common result is fainting, which can have tragic consequences. Remember, you're running on hard asphalt or even harder concrete. One runner I know passed out and hit his head near the finish of a hot weather half marathon. He is now permanently paralyzed.

The optimal temperature to run a marathon is around 40 degrees, but most of the largest marathons and half marathons in the United States are run in more temperate weather because warmer weather increases participation.

As a result, it's becoming increasingly common for marathon temperatures to top 70 degrees. In the 2012 Boston Marathon, over 2,100 runners were treated for heat exhaustion, dehydration, and other ailments as temperatures topped 80 degrees. And that's only the runners who were officially treated by medical personnel. *The untold story is how many of these runners suffered long-term damage to their heart, liver, kidneys, or brain.*

Years ago when I was young and stupid, I lost 12 pounds in a hot weather marathon. *I would never do it again.* There will always be another marathon. You only have one heart. Do not run marathons in hot weather.

167. Keep a Journal

A journal can help you keep track of your running progress, achievements, or interesting things you saw while running. Today, many runners use online journals that automatically upload workouts from their Garmins or apps that track their workouts.

I've tried a few, but I keep going back to my old school journal, which predates apps. Heck, it even predates computers!

A journal is also a great way to capture memories. Just to pick a day, I went to January 1, 1991 in my journal and found these remarks. *It was too icy to run on the highways, so Terry, Steve and I ran 6 miles on the Offutt Air Force Base perimeter road. I wore Asics shoes with hex screws as ice cleats. My knees were a little sore afterwards.* Every run that month was below 20 degrees. Later that month, one my friends would slip on the ice and dislocate his shoulder. Reading my journal, I can recall that day as if it were yesterday.

168. Use Caution with Music

Inevitably, some of your runs will be alone. Unless you're creative, recovery days can turn into just slogging in the miles—not fun. So, what can you do to make these recovery days more productive and enjoyable?

Perhaps the most popular approach is to listen to music. Many runners select music specifically because the tempo suits their running pace. Ask some fellow runners, and you'll find a surprising variety of music to suit every possible taste.

Listening to music helps the time fly by, but it also increases the risk of danger from inattention to your surroundings: cyclists, texting drivers, drunk drivers, muggers, potholes in the road, and so on. For these reasons, I never listen to music while running, but if you choose to do so, be very attentive to your surroundings.

Bonus Tip: "If you run with an iPod, rather than have the wires running down inside your shirt and hanging on everything, you can roll the wires around the iPod and place it inside your cap after you put the earbuds in. No wires anywhere!"—Charlie T

169. Set Goals for Motivation

Goals can give you the motivation to run on those days when it is so easy to come up with excuses not to run. It's too cold; it's too hot; it's too inconvenient; you're tired.

A friend of mine is on a "streak"—consecutive days of running every day. There's no competitive advantage to streaks, but it's a way to ensure he doesn't skip running on those dreary winter days.

It's so easy to let other events in our hectic day-to-day lives take priority over running. One day off becomes two and then three. Almost without noticing it, you haven't run in a week. Setting goals keeps you accountable and motivated to run.

Another way to add a little more zest to your running is to set goals that have nothing to do with speed or performance. Several of my friends are have a goal of running marathons in all 50 states or running 100 marathons. One ran 52 marathons in 52 weeks! That doesn't sound like fun to me, but whatever floats your boat.

Of course, it's not necessary for goals to be only racing events or times. Some of the unusual goals I've set over the years were to run part of the Western States 100-mile course, to run a race on a beach, and to run across the Golden Gate Bridge. Two of my friends ran the Great Wall of China Marathon.

170. Set Short-term Running Goals

You probably already have a long-term goal—run a marathon or run your next race faster than your last one. That's great! But a problem with long-term goals is that they can be so many months away they can take a back seat to day-to-day activities or unforeseen events that arise to divert your attention.

Short-term goals provide important day-to-day accountability.

Short-term goals solve that problem by giving you something to accomplish today or within the next week. My friend's goal of running every day provides him that short-term motivation. Your short-term goals might include "run at least 35 miles this week" or "run 100 miles this month."

Goals aren't just for races. I set goals for workouts and run the same workout every month or so to see how my training is progressing.

171. Use These Tips as Goals

Why not use some of the tips in this book as goals? You've probably seen several ideas you really like, but let's be honest, we're all so busy in our day-to-day lives that it's easy to forget to apply what we've learned. For example, you might set a goal to practice one of the speed tips, do the Billat 30-30 workout, or make your own orthotics.

172. Have a Post-Race Goal

Many runners and even some veterans go into a major race without having a post-event goal. Without follow-up goals, a post-race letdown can occur after the initial euphoria subsides, even if you meet your initial goal.

I believe this is why some novices drift away from running after finishing their first marathon. They see the marathon as one of the dozens of items on their bucket list to be checked off rather than starting a lifelong hobby.

They never realize that by finishing a marathon they had mastered one of the greatest antiaging secrets in the world—running—and instead, they let it slip away.

Post-race goals can help prevent drifting away from a lifelong healthy hobby.

Setting post-race goals can avoid the directionless letdown after reaching a major running milestone and help you make running a healthy lifelong activity.

Your post-race goal could be a destination run, improving your time, or running a different event. It doesn't have to be a big goal, just something to keep you involved in running. If you're racing for time, your goal might be to run faster in your next race.

173. Give Yourself a Reward

On those days when it's hard to get out the door—and even veterans have those days— reward yourself for completing the workout. The reward might be socializing with friends after the run, but feel free to give yourself more material rewards. You're improving your health. You're reducing your long-term medical expenses. Running is your investment in good health. You deserve a reward!

Running rewards are cheaper than heart surgery!

You might say, "If I run today, I will reward myself with a microbrew, a movie, or a new running top." Do whatever it takes for you. A heart bypass surgery from years of a sedentary lifestyle can cost over $50,000, not to mention the lost time at work and lost quality of life. If you look at rewards that way, a few dollars to keep you motivated to run is money well spent.

174. Set Cross Training Goals

Most runners have running goals, but even many veterans approach cross-training in a haphazard manner. Cross training can help reduce injuries and make you a better runner, so don't neglect cross-training goals.

For example, you might set goals for elliptical, cycling, swimming, or spinning. You could set goals for calories burned or percent body fat. My training partner has a goal of doing 500 calories of exercise every day. She uses an iWatch to track calories. In the next tip, you'll learn how setting cross-training goals helped me set a new state record in the 200m.

175. Hidden Value of Goal Setting

Whether you succeed or fail on the road to your goal, you can still learn a lot from the journey itself. Sometimes, these lessons can be even more valuable than achieving the original goal.

In 2016, my goals were to medal in the 200m and 400m at the USATF Indoor Masters Championships. Since I'd never raced the 200m seriously, I was shocked to see how muscular these national caliber sprinters were when compared to my skinny distance running peers. I finished 2nd in the 400m, but I failed to medal in the 200m, finishing fourth in 29.97. As a result of that failure, I realized that I'd have to reshape my body to the more muscular physique of a sprinter to be competitive in the 200m.

I had dabbled in weightlifting in the past, but now I resolved to set up a specific cross-training plan.

In 2017, I set a goal of lifting 4 million pounds. I fell short, but having a goal created structure, which led to hiring a personal trainer, finding specific muscle imbalances, and starting exercises to correct them. As a result, *I'm far stronger now than before I set this goal, even though I failed to reach the goal itself.*

Goals can be beneficial even if you fail to reach them.

The structured weightlifting plan made my normally fragile legs bulletproof. I ran injury free for the next year, running faster at age 70 than at 68, an almost unheard-of achievement at this level of competition. My speed improved in the 50, 100, 200, 400, and 800m events. Fifteen months later, I ran the 200m 0.88 seconds faster at 29.09 and set a new M70 state record.

Had it not been for the lessons learned from my failures, I might never have learned the tremendous benefits of weightlifting for older runners. More importantly, you would not have the opportunity to benefit from what I learned in Chapter 21 "Weightlifting for Masters Runners." Not a bad outcome for a failure!

That's the often overlooked secret to goal setting. Even if you don't achieve your goal, you can gain valuable wisdom from the journey.

18

Money Saving Tips

Running is one of the least expensive of all sports. Still, the cost of shoes, tops, shorts, physical therapy, massage therapy, out of pocket medical expenses, race registration, hotels, car rentals, and airfare to distant marathons can certainly add up. I have friends who fly to several marathons each year. Their expenses can easily top $1,000 per marathon. Multiply that by their goal of running a marathon in every state—or running 100 marathons—and you're looking at tens of thousands of dollars.

The good news is you can dramatically reduce these expenses. My current New Balance running shoes cost $43. My orthotics cost less than a quarter. My running shorts and tops cost less than $15 apiece, and my technical socks cost $2. My airfare to most national championships is free. Plus, over the years, I've saved hundreds of dollars in physical therapist expenses and out of pocket rehab costs by following the tips you'll learn in this chapter.

Now, we've covered some of these tips earlier, but this chapter consolidates them into one chapter for easy referral later. Plus, you'll get more detail on how to use each of these tips. Just consider this chapter as a thank you from the author for buying this book.

176. Shoes

Shoes are the most expensive piece of running apparel with some shoes costing over $150. I typically buy running shoes from a local running store, but once I know what works for me, I watch for sales and stock up. This works even better when stores sell their old models on clearance. I like buying last year's model because there are enough online reviews to find every problem with the shoe. If reviews say the shoe runs narrow and you have a wide foot, you can eliminate it from your search.

For example, I saw reviews that Hoka shoes helped runners with foot injuries and wondered if they might help rehab my chronic heel injury. They did help my injury, but the Clifton didn't fit me in other ways. When I found the Hoka Huaka on sale, I gave them a try. They were exactly what I needed. My local running store didn't have them, so I bought four pairs on clearance for $42 from Running Warehouse, saving over $300 off retail for the four pair of shoes.

A couple of years later after reading many positive reviews for the New Balance Zante v3, I bought a pair on clearance for $67. I liked them, so I bought another pair later on final clearance for only $42.

177. Socks

On a typical long run, your feet hit the ground about 10,000 times. What directly touches your foot on each of those 10,000 steps? Your socks. Even great shoes can cause problems without the right pair of socks, so you don't want to skimp on socks. Conversely, you don't want to overpay either. I typically pay less than two dollars a pair.

I buy most of my socks from TJ Maxx. They carry several major running brands—Nike, Adidas, RBX, Puma, Under Armour, Fila—as well as some off brands that are equally serviceable for running.

178. Tops and Shorts

I've bought some nice, inexpensive tops and shorts at TJ Maxx, Academy Sports, Target, and Walmart. One trick is to buy shorts without liners and then wear technical briefs under them, as I explained in an earlier chapter. This gives you a lot more options for running shorts. I especially like that I can buy a heavier material for winter running since most running shorts are tissue-paper thin.

179. Travel

I use a Southwest Airlines Rapid Rewards credit card for all my purchases, which accumulates enough points to pay for two or three round-trip flights each year. This year, I'll use points to fly free to the USATF Indoor and Outdoor Masters Championships. In the past three years, I've saved about $3,000 by using frequent flyer miles. There are other frequent flyer credit cards if Southwest does not fly into your nearest airport. If you plan to fly to several destination marathons in the coming years, this tip could save you thousands of dollars.

It's also a good idea to book everything months in advance. You can always cancel. If you wait until the last minute, airfares can double, and the flights you want might not be available.

180. Hotel and Car Rental

I usually travel with friends to races so we can split the cost of hotel rooms and car rentals. I get an additional discount on car rental by using USAA, although you can get discounts through numerous other sources, such as AAA, AARP, AMAC, and so on.

Sometimes I book my hotel through Hotwire since I don't care where I stay as long as it is a nice place. Even though you don't know the name of the hotel until after you book it, you can see the previous guests' ratings of the hotel. I prefer to stay in places with at least an 85% positive rating. You can also limit the choices to a certain section of the city—

Southeast, for example. Sometimes, you can guess the name of the hotel because there may only be one 3 ½ star hotel in that section.

If the ratings of available hotels are low or for some reason I want to stay in a specific hotel, I'll call the hotel directly, tell them the rates I've found online, and ask for their rates. Usually, I can come close to the Hotwire price, plus by dealing directly with the hotel, the reservation is cancellable up to the last minute if I find a better deal later.

181. Therapy

Physical therapy can be expensive and time-consuming. I use PTs occasionally, but I try to save time and money by following these steps.

a) Stop at the first sign of injury to keep it from getting worse.

b) Identify the cause of the injury and correct it.

c) Learn basic physical therapy for the injury.

I have three foam rollers, a Roll Recovery R8, an Interferential TENS unit, two heating pads, therapy balls, bands and several other therapy tools. That might sound like a lot, but my total cost for everything was only $300—roughly the cost of only three visits with a physical therapist. This equipment, plus equipment at my fitness center, gives me the ability to do almost all the exercises I would do at a therapist's office.

Don't get me wrong. I also use physical therapists. They can be great, but my first course of action is usually to see if I can manage rehab on my own. A variation of this might be to go to the PT a couple of times to learn what needs to be done and then do it myself at home. This not only saves money—it saves the travel time to and from the therapist. It also lets me do my rehab when it fits my schedule—in the evening, for example—rather than being forced to block time out of my workday when the therapist is available.

182. Orthotics

I haven't bought custom orthotics in many years, so I did an online search to determine the current. I wasn't too surprised to discover that custom orthotics can cost $300 to $500.

Not only do I save over $300 when I make my own orthotics, but I also don't have to go through the hassle of finding a shoe that works with a commercial orthotic. I can buy a shoe I like and modify its insert for my foot.

Even if you already have orthotics, they might not fit well when you buy new shoes, since your new shoes might have a different camber, heel-to-toe drop, or internal arch support. Ideally, you would get new orthotics every time you changed shoes, but that would get expensive.

Once you get the hang of it, your homemade orthotics can fit as well as the commercial version. Plus, it's so easy to make orthotics you can make a separate pair of all of your shoes, so you don't have to hassle with switching orthotics from one shoe to another.

183. Miscellaneous

I'm rough on sunglasses, but that no longer matters because my current pair cost only $39 online through Zenni Optical. I have a second, wider pair for cycling.

Of course, I only save a few dollars on my elastic laces, but even if they were more expensive, I'd still make them because they are far superior to the commercial version. More important, they help reduce lace-related injuries and the subsequent costs associated with recovery from those injuries.

Using tips in this chapter over the past five years I've saved over $1,000 in orthotics, $1,000 in shoes, $2,000 in hotels, $600 in car rentals, $600 in apparel, $200 in sunglasses, and over $3,000 in airfare. That's over $8,400—nearly $1,700 per year.

And that doesn't count how much I've saved by doing some of my own physical therapy. I have a friend who spends two hours each week with a physical therapist. Granted, she is a national caliber runner, and she can afford it, but that expense would be prohibitive for most runners unless it's covered by insurance.

19

Advice for Masters Runners

Masters runners face a different set of challenges. With age, runners tend to slow down. It takes longer to recover from injuries. Here are some secrets I've learned in decades of running since becoming a masters runner.

184. Injured? Don't Give Up. Seek State-of-the-Art Therapies

My advice to all runners is to be proactive when it comes to sports injuries. If your doctor says there's no cure or treatment for what ails you, do not give up! Your doctor might not be aware of state-of-the-art therapies for your condition, or your doctor might not mention a treatment because their facility is unable to provide it

If your injury isn't responding to conventional treatment, take charge of your health—don't just passively accept that you can't find a treatment. This is especially important for older runners who take even longer to recover from common running injuries.

Many veteran runners are leery of doctors, understandably since the typical physician's response to a running injury is, "Don't run on it for X number of weeks." Veteran runners have already tried taking time off, and it didn't work.

When your doctor is no help, ask other runners where they go for state-of-the-art medical care. My running friends have benefitted from new methods you might not be aware of—prolotherapy, platelet-rich plasma injections, interferential TENS stimulation with dry needling, active release therapy, and more.

Even though insurance might not cover some of these therapies, they aren't outrageously expensive.

In my case, I had a very severe case of plantar fasciitis in the heel. My general practitioner half-heartedly suggested a cortisone injection, but we both knew such injections weren't always successful. Worse, they could cause complications. Asking around among my running friends, I discovered a sports therapist who did interferential TENS therapy with dry needling. In three treatments over two weeks, the injury was 90% cured. I was so amazed at the speed of recovery that I bought my own inferential TENS unit. Some of my running friends have had success with prolotherapy, another treatment that's not typically covered by insurance.

If you have a serious injury and it is not responding to conventional treatment, or you've been told that you can never run again, consider these steps.

Get a second opinion. This is important for all major illnesses, not just running injuries. My mother-in-law was diagnosed with lung cancer. We flew her to a state-of-the-art hospital where they successfully killed the tumor with only four noninvasive treatments over the course of two weeks. That was over a decade ago. Had we passively accepted her first doctor's diagnosis, she'd likely be dead today.

Ask runners for referrals. This is how I have found almost all my successful interventions. If there is a major sports team in your area, ask what specialists they use. I've suffered through injuries for months that were resolved in only a couple of sessions when treated by the right sports medicine specialist.

Try alternative therapies. This is so important that I've expanded on it in the next tip.

185. Consider Alternative Therapies

If you have exhausted your options in conventional medicine, don't give up until you've considered alternative therapies that have worked for other runners. Sadly, I have friends with career-threatening injuries who refuse to consider alternative therapies, which means they may never run at the same level again.

Here's my take on alternative medicine. The medical community can be painfully slow in accepting new approaches to old problems. For example, chelation therapy, which was widely denounced three decades ago, is now a mainstream medical treatment for some types of cancer.

Still, alternative therapies don't work for everyone. They often have a relatively high failure rate, which is one reason why they still fall into the alternative category. This doesn't mean they're worthless. It means that you may have to try more than one strategy to find something that works for you.

For illustration purposes, let's assume that the success rate for all alternative therapies is 15%. (Again, this is purely a hypothetical percentage.) The probability that your first alternative approach will succeed is only 15%, but with each subsequent attempt with a new alternative therapy, your odds improve. On the second approach, the odds increase to 28%; on the third attempt, the odds increase to 39%; and on the fourth attempt, odds increase to 48% and so on. Of course, there is always a possibility there is nothing you can do for your injury. My point is you won't know until you try.

Today's alternative therapy might be tomorrow's mainstream medicine. Profiling is a good example. Rather than using the conventional one-size-fits-all approach to cancer treatment, scientists now look at genetic profiles to determine which conventional treatment is best-suited for each patient. A couple of decades ago, cancer profiling would have been considered quackery.

The bottom line is that if your doctor says there's no cure for your injury, don't give up. I was told by two doctors at the Mayo Clinic in 1999 that I could never run again. Since then, I've run over 15,000 miles and set multiple state records and one world record.

Your doctor might not be aware of alternative therapies or might not be willing to risk a malpractice lawsuit to recommend them. Even doctors who do believe in alternative therapies might not be able to discuss them with you because of the rules imposed on them by their regulating agencies.

It's your life and health. Be proactive. Research your options, including alternative therapies. You make the final decision.

186. Cross-training—Yes or No?

Some runners swear by cross training, while old-school runners are equally vociferous that time spent cross-training could be better utilized by just running more miles. Here's my take.

Cross-training is a great way to add strength and flexibility while recovering from the previous day's hard run, but the risk of injury from some types of cross training is too high if you are serious about running. Looking back over the years, about half of my injuries came from cross-training.

For competitive runners, the ideal cross-training should be low-impact, but specific to the strength, range of motion, or endurance you need to become a better runner.

Over half of my injuries came from cross training.

The best cross-training exercises are bicycling, spinning, swimming, aqua jogging, elliptical, Stairmaster, and cross-country skiing. Weightlifting is also excellent if you learn proper form and recover enough between sets to ensure you maintain excellent form. In my opinion, older runners should avoid complex lifts that require multiple movements, such as Olympic lifts. They increase the risk of injury while not adding a commensurate increase in benefits compared to simple movement lifts.

Personally, I have found that timed exercises—rushing through one exercise to another as fast as possible—is a prescription for injury for me because eventually, my form gets sloppy. Poor form increases the risk of injury.

Competitive runners should avoid high-risk cross-training.

Bonus Tip: Runners possess very strong muscles and tendons for linear motion, but the tendons and muscles used for lateral motion and extended range of motion are much weaker. That's why runners, especially older runners, have a high risk of injury when they first start doing high impact cross-training, like bench jumps, burpees, Olympic lifts, and similar exercises. It's important to be conservative at first. Your strong running muscles can create a false sense of how much you can lift or how many reps you can do. It's easy to strain the weaker muscles and tendons.

It comes down to this—why are you running? If getting faster is unimportant and you're running mostly to stay fit and lose weight, then disregard my comments about high-risk cross-training. Yes, it might not make you a better runner, but so what? Running is just one of the things you're doing to stay fit and trim. In organized fitness classes you can get fit, look better, lose weight, socialize, and have a great time. I love my organized fitness classes, but since I'm a competitive runner, I was very careful to choose a club that allowed me to modify some of the lifts so I could focus my workout on my ultimate goal—becoming a better runner.

187. What About Yoga?

Yoga is fine, but if you're a competitive runner, never lose sight of your primary objective. Your goal for yoga is not to get better at yoga—you will, of course, but that's not your goal—your goal is to use yoga to become a better runner.

It is critical not to lose sight of the big picture. *You are a runner, not a human pretzel.* You do not need to be as flexible as your instructor to be a better runner or to reduce running injuries. You should not attempt to do the extreme movements of your instructor or advanced students in your class.

As a runner, your muscles are always going to be tighter than those of someone who only practices yoga. You do not need their range of motion to excel in running. What you need is muscular balance and dynamic stretching of muscles that are tightened from running. I find it more efficient to incorporate a few yoga exercises into my weightlifting warm-up and cool down program rather than spend an entire hour doing yoga.

188. Reconsider Marathon Training

It pains me to write this as the target market for this book is predominantly marathoners and half marathoners, but it's something older runners should know. Competitive marathoning can be detrimental to your long-term health if you're over 50.

Let's be clear. I'm not talking to the vast majority of readers. I'm talking to those runners who put in high miles for months at a time to competitively race the marathon distance.

Long duration exercise floods the body with byproducts of energy production—especially free radicals and cortisol. Without sufficient recovery time, cortisol and free radical levels will remain high, never recovering to normal levels. Over time, this can suppress your immune system. This is especially true for older adults.

My circle of friends includes several older marathoners who have run fast enough to qualify for the Boston marathon. When I look this group, I see a disproportionate number of diseases that have been linked to a weak immune system.

Among these dozen or so marathoners, two have cancer, two have hypothyroidism, one has heart disease, one has Graves' disease, and one has diabetes. Free radicals and high cortisol levels have been linked to all of these diseases.

What do these serious runners have in common? They're all over the age of 50, they all train much harder than recreational runners, and they put in high mileage month after month.

In 1999, I had blood tests done by an anti-aging clinic that compared my blood chemistry to that of a cross-section of the population. When I sat down to talk with the doctor, his first question was, "What in the world have you been doing?" He explained that my blood chemistry was that of a 35-year-old (I was 51 at the time), but that my free radical levels were those of a 72-year-old!

I had gone for a hard 14-mile run the previous day. Even though it was 24 hours later, my body was still suffering from the flood of toxins into my system.

That was a wake-up call for me. I stopped marathon training almost immediately. I still do long runs, but I take at least two days of easy recovery afterward. I also take vitamins to reduce free radicals and cortisol.

Yet changing running habits can be very hard for some runners. Another old friend died because he refused to quit training at a very high level after being diagnosed with cancer. He even attempted an ultramarathon less than one week after surgery. I privately told him that he needed to reduce his running until his body could heal, but he chose his own path.

Let me be clear. Recreational marathoners who run 25 to 30 miles a week and run the occasional marathon shouldn't worry. As a marathoner, your health risk is still far less than that of nonrunners. Plus, it's not the marathon itself that raises your potential health risks. The marathon will be over in a few hours. Instead, it's the years of high mileage training that creates chronically high cortisol and free radical levels without sufficient recovery time to flush those toxins out of the body.

Marathon training stresses the immune system. Eat healthily, take supplements, and get enough recovery between hard workouts.

---

189. Compete in Senior Olympics

In 1996, I headed to my local track for a workout, only to find it filled with an amazing sight—silver-haired men and women running, jumping, and throwing in what appeared to be a high-level track meet. When I asked what was going on, an official told me it was the state finals of the Senior Olympics. As I watched, I was inspired by these healthy seniors. I vowed to run in the Senior Olympics even though I had never run track in my life.

Fast forward 20 years, I'm currently the Tennessee Senior Games state champion in every running event in my age group, but that's not why I participate. I participate to stay young, to have fun, and to inspire my nonrunning friends to get off the sofa and start exercising.

Try it. There are lots of sports besides running: golf, basketball, volleyball, tennis, swimming, cycling, and more. Go to www.nsga.com to find senior games near you.

20

How to Slow Aging

Twenty years ago, my 400m and 800m times were unimpressive. Today, my times are a little slower, but I have slowed far less than my competition. In 2016, I ran one of the top 20 times in the world for the indoors 400m. I've been ranked as high as #11 in the world in the indoor 800m. Let me stress that I have not gotten faster. I've slowed down, but *I've slowed less than my competition.* In effect, I've slowed the aging process. So can you.

One of my friends is one of the world's top anti-aging scientists. He and his fellow researchers believe we will be able to dramatically slow or even stop aging within the next 20 years. He views aging as a disease and believes we will eventually find a cure. Once that happens, your life expectancy would only be limited by accidents, trauma, or rare illnesses.

It's easy to be skeptical, but I've spent many hours talking with him about antiaging advances that aren't being reported by the media—mostly because they are too complex to cover in a 60-second news spot. We're not talking about merely curing cancer or heart disease. Instead, these advances would replace aging heart cells with youthful cells that would be strong enough to resist cancer naturally.

Antiaging advances will change the world, but they might not trickle down to us for another 20 years. Fortunately, there are steps you can take right now to slow how fast your body is aging.

190. You Can Slow the Aging Process

How did I go from being only a little better than a mid-pack runner to being world ranked? Well, I certainly didn't do it based solely on talent. It came from two very important factors.

a. I immersed myself in everything I could learn about running, racing, and recovery. Many of those tips I'm sharing with you in this book.

b. I aged slower than my competition.

A couple of decades ago, I attended a talk by Walter Bortz M.D., author of *Dare to Be 100*. According to Dr. Bortz, adults begin to lose "vitality" at a rate of 2% per year starting at age 30. Once vitality drops to 20%, they would begin to suffer serious and even life-threatening illnesses.

Dr. Bortz found that exercise, diet, and lifestyle changes could slow the rate of decline to 1/2% a year. Thus, 30-year-olds have a choice— they can neglect their health and reach the critical level of 20% vitality at age 70, or they can take proactive steps to age slower, reaching age 70 with 80% of their vitality still intact.

Interestingly, Dr. Bortz is also a runner and veteran of 35 marathons including the Boston Marathon in 2005. His webpage indicates that at age 81, he still runs 16 miles week. It's great to see someone who practices what he preaches.

Years later, as I was recovering from an injury that doctors had told me would end my running career, I recalled Dr. Bortz' words. At age 53, I could never regain the performances of my youth, but I might catch my competition by aging slower. I resolved to learn all I could about slowing the aging process and apply those steps to my life.

Today, it's not uncommon to meet people I haven't seen in years who comment on how young and healthy I look. That's not genetics or luck. I work every day to stay as young as possible for as long as possible.

Slowing the aging process will not result in immediate performance gains, but that's not its purpose. Instead, you'll see those gains slowly over the years as you age slower than your peers.

191. Importance of Nutrition and Supplements

Good nutrition and supplements are the foundation for staying as young and healthy as possible. Many nutritionists believe the average person can get all the vitamins and supplements they need by eating a healthy diet. I'm skeptical, but even if that were true, you're far from the "average" person. As a runner, you'll run further in one training run than the average person runs in their entire adult lifetime, yet your Recommended Daily Allowance (RDA) is the same.

That doesn't make sense. Obviously, you're expending far more energy, and as a result, you'll need far more nutrients than the average person.

Plus, RDA is the minimum level of vitamins required to prevent disease. That's *not* your goal! Fitness is not just the absence of disease; it's maintaining energy, alertness, and vitality in our daily lives. You're not just trying to prevent scurvy, for goodness sakes, you're trying to stay active, vital, and youthful for as long as possible!

Studies show distance running floods the body with free radicals and other byproducts of energy production. Studies have linked energy byproducts to many major illnesses, including arteriosclerosis, COPD, heart disease, cancer, diabetes, and impairment of the immune system. It's important to get enough nutrients daily to combat these toxic byproducts of exercise.

Twenty years ago, I attended a speech given by Dr. Kenneth Cooper author of *The Antioxidant Revolution*. Cooper's premise was that running conveys enormous health benefits up to about 12 miles per week. Then, health risks stay about the same until 30 miles per week when risk begins to increase once again. The resulting chart looked like a ski jump—much higher on the sedentary side than on the extreme running side, with a low point in the middle between 12 to 30 miles per week.

Dr. Cooper believes even though runners have lower than average risk, they could reduce their risk even further by dropping down to 12 miles per week or taking supplements to reduce the risk from these oxidative stresses at higher exercise levels.

Dr. Cooper caught a lot of flak for this controversial position at the time, but to me his message was clear. Running significantly reduces the risk of major illnesses. Although risk begins to tick upwards again at higher exercise levels, this slight uptick can be countered with supplements to reduce oxidative stress.

There was another interesting takeaway from Dr. Cooper's chart. There was no specific mileage at which risk began to increase again. It was a gradual curve somewhere between 12 and 30 miles per week.

I believe this is because each runner has their unique tipping point— the point at which the body can no longer keep up with the damage caused by chronically high levels of cortisol and oxidative stress. There are lots of variables affecting this tipping point—sleep, stress, diet, volume and intensity of mileage, cross-training, age, and the simple fact that each person's body reacts differently to exercise and oxidative stresses.

It also stands to reason that runners would have higher nutritional needs than the average non-running population. For older runners, it could be even higher, because as we age, *our cells become less efficient in utilizing the nutrients in our food. To compensate, the prudent approach would be to flood your body with enough nutrients to ensure that it always has enough raw materials to recover from your workouts.*

I take about a dozen supplements a day. Skeptics might see it as a waste of money. I see it as health insurance. I used to get sick every winter. When I started taking vitamins, the number of days lost to these illnesses dropped dramatically. I strongly believe that supplements have made a difference in my life.

192. Bioidentical Hormone Replacement for Women

Fourteen years ago, my wife had a total hysterectomy. She went from premenopausal to postmenopausal overnight, yet she didn't suffer any of the common symptoms of menopause. That's because, at her request, the doctor prescribed bioidentical hormone replacement (BIHR) therapy instead of traditional hormone replacement therapy.

One and a half decades later, BIHR still isn't mainstream, but it should be. Instead of replacing one or two hormones, the bioidentical approach replaces three or more major chemicals that decrease dramatically after menopause. Further, the ratio and amount of these hormones can be adjusted individually for each woman.

Some doctors point out that BIHR therapy has not been proven in clinical trials, but that's because the therapy cannot be tested using traditional FDA methods. Since the ratios vary individually, each participant would be receiving different amounts of the hormones being tested. Thus, it would be impossible to do double-blind clinical trials to prove conclusively that BIHR therapy is better than traditional hormone replacement therapy.

Fortunately, women don't need a double-blind clinical trial to find out what works for them. All they need to do is try it for themselves. What's more, most insurance carriers will cover BIHR prescriptions. When I mention BIHR therapy to women runners, I get one of two responses. They've never heard of it, or they've tried it and love it.

193. Hormone Boosting for Men

By age 50, male testosterone levels drop significantly. By age 70, T levels drop by more than half. It's hard to listen to sports radio without hearing an ad for a "Low T" clinic. Still, I'm not a fan of hormone replacement for men because it tricks the body into thinking it's producing enough hormones, so the body's natural hormone producing factories shut down. There are also studies that indicate it might increase the risk of cancer.

For most runners ages 50 and up, a better approach than low T drugs is to increase the body's natural ability to produce testosterone by high-intensity exercise, such as the HIIT workouts we'll discuss later in this chapter. High-intensity exercise boosts the body's hormone-producing factories for several hours.

You can further help that process along by ensuring the body's factories have enough raw materials to make hormones. Since these cellular factories become less efficient with age, supplementing your diet with certain nutrients is a good idea. Specifically, that would be amino acids, such as whey protein powder. In summer, I end almost every day with a protein smoothie made with almond milk, ice cubes, chocolate whey protein powder, and frozen strawberries or bananas.

194. Manage Your Stress

Stress floods the body with cortisol. To a degree, this is a good thing because it preps the body for the flight or fight syndrome by temporarily shutting down energy going to unnecessary systems, like digestion or the immune system. Unfortunately, when cortisol levels get high and stay there due to constant stress, it can damage the immune system. That, in turn, leads to increased risk of colds, flu, cancer, heart disease, pneumonia, and a myriad of other diseases.

Fortunately, moderate exercise reduces stress. Runners should be able to manage stress without prescription drugs.

195. Importance of Sleep

Your body uses the time you are asleep to heal itself and boost hormone levels. Sleep also boosts your immune system.

I avoid prescription sleeping pills because they don't create the deep REM sleep your body needs. Instead, I take melatonin and valerian root every night about 20 minutes before bedtime. Valerian root is a natural, mild sleeping aid, like chamomile tea. Melatonin is produced naturally by the body to aid sleep, but melatonin levels decline with age.

I will sometimes take a nap if I feel tired after a hard workout.

196. Importance of Weight Management

Statistically, being overweight increases the risk of virtually all the diseases of seniors. Obesity—about 50 pounds overweight for women and 60 pounds for the average height man—doubles the risk of heart disease and cancer. It more than triples the risk of diabetes and Alzheimer's Disease.

Medicare costs for obese seniors are over 60% higher than seniors who are not overweight. Merely being overweight doesn't necessarily reduce your life expectancy, but it can reduce your quality of life in your senior years by increasing the risk of many debilitating diseases.

I weigh within 10 pounds of what I weighed when I graduated from college nearly 50 years ago.

197. HIIT— High-Intensity Interval Training

High-intensity interval training is one of the best training tips I can share with older runners. Studies show that after very high-intensity short duration efforts, testosterone levels, and human growth hormone increase significantly. These two hormones are essential to healthy aging and optimal running performance.

Years before it became the rage, I was doing variations of HIIT taught by my friend Phil Campbell, author of *Ready Set Go Fitness*.

Here are some of my favorite HIIT workouts.

a. 6-8 reps of 10 seconds all-out sprints
b. 6-8 reps of 10 seconds of hill sprints
c. Eight reps of 20 seconds of air squats with a 10-second recovery between sets
d. Three sets of various weightlifts to exhaustion in each set

HIIT also speeds up the metabolism, so if you're running to lose weight, adding high-intensity cross training would be a real asset. There are some caveats for older runners. You'll find them in the weightlifting chapter.

198. Importance of Attitude

In addition to the steps already mentioned, older runners need to quit thinking of themselves as "old." Attitude is critically important to staying young. You need to delete from your vocabulary phrases like "I'm not getting any younger" and "What can I expect at my age." You need to delete words like geezer, old fart, or old man from your vocabulary. Interestingly, older women don't do this nearly as much. Guys should follow their lead.

Attitude is critical to staying young. Years ago, I went to see a doctor with a pain in my right knee. After some tests, he said it was probably arthritis and shrugged, "It's pretty normal at your age." I laughed, "My left knee is the same age, and it doesn't have arthritis!" I immediately resolved to find another doctor. That was 20 years ago—I'm still running.

The moral of the story is that when you have a pain or an injury, take proactive steps to fix it. See your doctor, see a specialist, see a chiropractor, or seek out alternative treatments. Don't stop until you find a solution.

Do _not_ just resign yourself to pain as an inevitable part of aging. Be proactive.

At the Huntsman World Games, I met several senior athletes who had been overweight or ill and had started exercising out of desperation or on their doctor's recommendation. These seniors are now active, healthy, and enjoying swimming, pickleball, volleyball, running, or other sports.

On the other hand, a few years back, I met a sickly-looking guy who appeared to be in his 70s. He complained to me about his many illnesses and told me his medications cost $5,000 a year out-of-pocket after his insurance. I was shocked to learn he was only 55 years old. He died a few months later.

Don't be like this man. It was too late for him, but you can push back against aging starting now. Resolve before you leave this page to do one thing to slow your aging process. It could be HIIT, supplements, weight management, or whatever sounds best to you. Resolve to fight aging starting right now.

The good news—great news actually—is that if you are out of shape, overweight, and in poor health, you might be able to reverse the effects of aging! If you follow social media, you'll see lots of exercise testimonials from seniors who couldn't walk up a set of stairs who are now as active and vital as they were 20 years ago. It's not too late!

21

Weightlifting for Masters Runners

M any years ago, I watched an older runner win every event in his age group in the state senior games. It left such an impression on me that I resolved to do it as well, but try as I might, I was never fast enough to be competitive in the short sprints.

Finally, upon moving into the M70 age group in 2017, I raced every running event in the Tennessee Senior Game Finals, winning all eight events from the 50m to the 10K. By the end of the week, I had also set four new state records in the 50, 200, 400, and 800-meter races—missing the 100m state record by only a quarter of a second. Only a few months earlier, I placed 2nd in the 400m at the National Senior Games. How did I improve so much in the sprints? Here are the secrets to my success.

   a) I added weightlifting to my weekly routine.

   b) I added fast, short intervals to my workouts.

   c) I avoided injury, which had frequently occurred in the past when I attempted high-speed training.

The real secret was weightlifting. When I added weightlifting three times a week to my training routine, my formerly fragile legs became almost bulletproof, allowing me to train without injury for months at a time. Equally important, this lack of injuries allowed me to do fast intervals.

As an added benefit, the lack of injuries allowed me to improve in longer events as well. Let's look at some benefits of weightlifting for age 50+ runners.

199. Weightlifting Boosts Testosterone Levels

By age 70, testosterone levels can decline by 50% or more. Studies show that high-intensity weightlifting boosts testosterone levels in older men. This is a very valuable benefit because testosterone not only boosts racing performance, it has many anti-aging benefits. This is especially important for distance runners because, in some cases, distance training reduces testosterone levels. At age 52, when I was training for a marathon, my testosterone had dropped to 235. In 2017 at age 70, it was 438. This is primarily due to stopping marathon training and adding HIIT (High-Intensity Interval Training) to my weekly routine. As you learned in the previous chapter, there are other ways to do HIIT, but weightlifting is easy and you can do it in the convenience of your own home.

200. Weightlifting Prevents Injuries

Another overlooked benefit of weightlifting is that it can reduce running injuries. Obviously, it does this by strengthening muscles and tendons, but there are even more benefits for older runners

On an autumn trail run, I tripped and fell hard. Usually, I just stumble to the ground, but this was a full face-plant. The force of the landing left me a bit dazed, but after getting up, I was surprised to discover no injuries. I had instinctively put out my hands to cushion my landing. A year earlier, I wouldn't have had the upper body strength to catch myself like that. Weightlifting had provided an unexpected benefit.

Weightlifting can help you improve as a masters runner, provided you use the right approach. Let's start with how to avoid some common weightlifting mistakes.

201. Avoid Poor Lifting Form

Weightlifting uses muscles you might not have used in years, so it's critically important to use proper form. I was fortunate to have an excellent coach to show me technique, but when I was lifting at home without supervision, I still managed to hurt myself. Proper form is even more important for masters runners because ligaments tend to become more brittle with age.

202. Avoid Too Much Too Soon

Runners have really strong muscles for straight ahead movement, but the lateral movement muscles are often very weak by comparison. This muscle imbalance can create the mistaken impression that you can lift more than you really can.

This "more is better" mentality can lead to injuries as runners attempt to do too much too soon.

203. Be Cautious with New Workouts

This was my worst mistake. We'd do a new workout, and I'd immediately test myself to see how much I could lift. It's a good idea to start out much lower than what you could probably lift when you first try a new movement. Until you've done the lift a few times, your form probably won't be right. Plus, it's easier to learn the proper lift technique if you use a lighter weight. Second, the weight or the range of motion might be too much for muscles that haven't been used in that manner.

204. Avoid "Racing" a Weight Workout

Timed workouts are a staple for some fitness centers. The goal is to race through a series of exercises—burpees, pull-ups, pushups, and so on—as fast as possible. There are some benefits to timed workouts, but I suggest older runners avoid them.

When you attempt to go from one exercise to another as quickly as possible, eventually you get tired. When you get tired, your form breaks down, which creates a high risk for injuries. This is especially true for older runners who tend to be less flexible and have more fragile legs.

To my knowledge, there is no research to prove your running will improve more by racing through a set of lifts than taking a few extra seconds to do the same exercises, but there is a great deal of anecdotal evidence to indicate that rushing lifts results in injuries.

In my opinion, it is far more important to make sure that your body is in the proper position before starting each lift and that you are recovered enough to perform the exercise using good form.

You can still do the individual exercises explosively. Just take an extra second or so to ensure you are using good form for the next rep.

205. Avoid Complex Movements

In our fitness center, we avoid timed exercises and lifts that require multiple, rapid movements, such as Olympic snatch or clean and jerk. Instead of the snatch, for example, we would do the movements separately—sets of deadlifts, barbell squats, and overhead presses.

Let me be clear. Complex movements can be great exercises. It's just that the risk of injury is much higher than doing each part of the exercise separately.

So, with these pitfalls out of the way, what exercises should you consider? There are many very good cross training exercises for runners. Rather than provide a definitive list, I'm going to list a few of my favorites.

206. Air Squats and Jump Squats

The air squat begins by standing erect with hands by your sides. Squat by bending at the knee until your thighs are parallel to the ground while simultaneously raising your arms straight in front of you. Reverse the movements to stand upright. If you've never done air squats, you might need to put one hand on a chair back or wall to help maintain your balance. Eventually, you should do this exercise without support because improving balance is part of this exercise. You can find lots of YouTube videos on air squats so I won't explain them further.

The next step is to do dumbbell squats. Just do a squat while holding dumbbells at your sides in each hand.

The next progression is the jump squat. A jump squat is simply an air squat done so forcefully your feet leave the ground. Jump squats should be done in sets of five with nearly full recovery between sets. If you can do far more than five jump squats, the next step is dumbbell jump squats. I'm currently doing three sets of 5 jump squats while holding two 40-pound dumbbells.

207. Bench Step Ups

Step up on a low bench with one leg. Tighten glutes to stand erect on the bench with one leg while raising the other leg into a running position with the knee bent at a 90-degree angle. Your arms should move the same as if you were running. Step down very slowly, perhaps to a 4-count. Repeat.

The next progression is to do step ups with dumbbells. You can also raise the bench higher. I find that a typical weight bench is too high for me, so I use a lower bench.

208. Wall Balls

This is one of my favorite exercises. Squat in front of a wall with a medicine ball held at your chest. Explosively stand up while pushing with both arms to throw the ball high against the wall. Catch the ball as it comes down. Immediately let the weight of the ball carry you down into the squat position. Repeat.

A variation of this exercise is to explosively jump so hard your feet leave the ground when throwing the ball. When doing this, just let the ball bounce when it comes down and catch it on the rebound. Reset your feet, squat, and repeat the jump and throw.

You should do both variations of this exercise. Each variation works the muscles differently.

209. Medicine Ball Routine

A strong core is important because it helps maintain good form when you are tired. It also improves breathing. You've probably seen runners who are hunched over as they run. When the body is hunched over, it compresses the diaphragm, which in turn limits the amount of oxygen your lungs can breathe in.

Medicine ball (med ball) exercises are a good way to build core strength. My routine includes V ups, med ball crunches, Russian Twists, and toe touches. These exercises focus on different areas of the ab-dominal muscles.

210. Glute Exercises

Glute exercises have become a bit of a fad among fitness advocates, but they can improve your running, especially if you want to run faster or have more power on hills.

My favorite glute exercises are air squats, jump squats, weighted walking lunges with a plate held overhead, single leg bridge (hip thrusts), Bulgarian squats, and single leg deadlifts.

211. Planks

Planks and plank variations are good ways to strengthen your core. The basic plank is supporting yourself with your forearms and toes on the ground while keeping your body straight. Don't let your hips sink or rise high in the air.

When I first started doing planks two years ago, I could barely hold this position for 20 seconds. After a year, I could hold the same position for 5 minutes.

22

Diet, Weight, and Nutrition

I debated on whether to include this chapter. After all, diet advice is everywhere. Worse, it's often conflicting advice. In the end, I decided it would be a disservice to readers to not at least share my thoughts on the subject.

The human body is a biomechanical machine and machines need the right fuel to operate at peak performance. Sure, some people might be able to eat junk food without any negative consequences for weeks, months, or even years, but eventually, that poor diet is going to come back to bite them.

As a result of sedentary lifestyles and poor eating habits, obesity has become an epidemic in America. One in three adults is obese—about 50 pounds or more overweight. Obesity increases medical expenses by over 60%. It increases the risk of breast cancer by up to 200%, heart disease by up to 100%, and diabetes by over 500%—that's right, 500%.

Perhaps of more immediate importance to you as a runner, extra pounds slow you down.

212. Every Pound Affects Running Performance

Specifically, every extra pound over your ideal weight slows your running performance by about 3 seconds per mile. For a runner who is 20 pounds overweight, that works out to nearly 3 minutes in a 5K and 12 minutes in a half marathon. This isn't an exact science, so if you're overweight, your benefit might be more or less if you lose weight, but you will be faster!

If you want to race faster, maintaining your ideal weight as your race date approaches can be critical to your race performance.

Case study: Based on years of personal experience, my ideal race weight is 132 pounds. Under that, I'm weaker. Over that, I'm slower, but it's very difficult for me to maintain weight at 132 pounds for more than a few weeks. Instead, I'll do what some elite athletes do. I'll allow myself to gain a few pounds during the off-season and then adjust my diet to get back to racing weight at least one month before the event itself. I've discovered that losing significant weight in the last couple of weeks prior to a race is counterproductive because it just makes me weaker.

Adjust your diet to reach your ideal weight at least one month before your major race.

---

213. Need Motivation to Lose Weight?

Of course, the hard part of losing weight is finding the motivation to do it. This can be really, really hard, but if you sincerely want to become a better runner, this simple exercise might provide all the motivation you need.

Fill a backpack with the amount of weight you want to lose and go for a run over one of your regular running routes. Even better, do some hill repeats.

Let's say you're 10 pounds overweight. It is amazing how hard it is to run uphill with a 10-pound backpack. Imagine how much faster you could run if you weren't carrying that extra weight.

214. Lose Weight and Reduce Injuries

Carrying extra weight also increases the risk of running injuries. Once you do the weighted backpack carry, you'll notice that not only does it require more effort, it changes your running form. It also puts a lot more pressure on your knees and arches. Those are just injuries waiting to happen until you lose weight.

215. Find the Diet that Works for You

I have friends who have resolved significant health problems after switching to a paleo diet. Sounds interesting, but wait! I also have friends who switched to a gluten-free diet and swear by its benefits. So, which one is the best? With so many different diets out there, how do you find one that's right for you?

In the second chapter of this book, you learned feet are like snowflakes—no two are exactly alike. Thus, it's difficult to find the perfect shoe. When it comes to diet, people are also like snowflakes. Your brother and sister might be able to drink milk all day long, while you inherited your great-grandfathers lactose intolerance. The diet that works for your friends might not be the best for you.

This leads to a good news/bad news situation. The bad news you already know. It's hard to find the perfect diet. In fact, it's so hard that many people just give up. The good news is that these people are wrong. A better diet exists for them—they just haven't found it yet.

It's not just a matter of how much you eat. It's what you eat, when you eat, and getting the right balance of carbs, proteins, and fats for your unique genetics and exercise level.

Case Study: Throughout most of my adult life, I would go through periods of being hungry followed by lethargy and irritability. At age 55, I discovered these were common symptoms of hypoglycemia—low blood sugar—and it was fairly common in my family tree. As a result, many of the common mantras about eating and running didn't work for me. Carbo-loading would create a quick burst of energy followed by a crash a couple of hours later. A high carbohydrate diet resulted in similar energy swings, so I went to more proteins and fats. Today, I carry high-protein energy bars with me wherever I go. It's not unusual for me to eat 4 to 6 times a day. On the other hand, one of my friends, a world-class runner, eats only once a day.

The bottom line is that you must figure out what works for you. No diet is likely to be perfect.

216. Avoid Artificial Sweeteners

Personally, I avoid all artificial sweeteners. I realize this is a bit controversial since 180 million Americans use artificial sweeteners every day, but they have some troubling side effects.

Studies show that frequent users of artificial sweeteners gain weight. Researchers are not sure why, but some studies have found that artificial sweeteners can increase cravings and glucose insensitivity. Some studies also report increased health risks of major diseases. Other studies have failed to confirm this correlation. To me, artificial sweeteners aren't worth the risk.

I use Stevia, a natural sweetener made from leaves of the Stevia plant. I just carry the packets with me in my gym bag.

23

Never Stop Learning

As I gathered data for this book, I'd ask my running friends—many of whom are world champions or Olympians—one question. "If you could share just one tip with other runners, what would it be?" I received some excellent answers. Be consistent. Avoid injuries. Put in the miles. Don't try to do too much too fast. Find a great coach. These bits of wisdom appeared many times—and with good reason. They are excellent advice.

My final bit of wisdom is a little different. You'll learn it soon, but first here is some background that helped form my philosophy about running.

217. It's Easy to Be Good

Whether it's life or running, it's relatively easy to be good at what you are doing—show up every day, be on time, be responsible, work hard, and do your job. It's just that easy, yet based on my multiple decades on this planet, millions of people never grasp this simple concept.

Woody Allen famously quipped, "Eighty percent of success is showing up." It's the same with running. Get a good training plan, show up every day, be responsible, and work hard. You will get better.

218. The Secret to Becoming the Best You Can Be

Ah, but to be great—to become the best you can be—that's another matter entirely.

To be great requires more than discipline. It requires more than just showing up and following a plan because thousands of your competitors are already doing that. You have to do more, but what should you do? Here's the secret. It's not just about logging more miles; it's about being smarter with your training.

Becoming great requires thinking, trying, doing, making mistakes, and learning from those mistakes.

Most important, becoming great requires you not only learn from your mistakes, you need to learn from the mistakes of others because life is too short to make all the mistakes you can possibly make in running. Trust me on this. I've been running for 40 years, and I still haven't made them all.

Throughout history, many people have risen to greatness by learning from the mistakes and successes of others and modeling themselves after highly successful people. They've also learned from books by icons like Dale Carnegie, Steven Covey, and Tony Robbins about the importance of finding a role model who is great at what you want to accomplish and then modeling your behavior after that person.

Sometimes, asking a question can provide great insight into whatever is troubling you. My Aunt Nell, a woman who made millions in real estate, used to tell me as a child, "If you ask a question, some people might think you're dumb for five minutes. But if you don't ask those questions, you could be dumb for the rest of your life!"

It's equally important to listen when someone offers constructive advice. I remember running with a younger runner who was complaining about a nagging injury that just wouldn't go away. I'd had this injury and knew immediately what he was doing wrong, but every time I tried to explain, he would cut me off to tell me more about the problem. After several attempts and getting cut off each time, I waited until the run was over and tried one more time.

Once again, he interrupted me. This time I abruptly cut him off, saying sharply, "I know how to treat this injury. Do you want to shut up and let me tell you how to treat it, or do you just want to hear yourself complain?" Blunt? Yes, but it worked.

Sometimes, we can all be like that runner. We get so focused on the problem and what didn't work that we fail to seek out experienced advice on what might work. Worse, we ignore advice when it's handed to us on a platter, as it was in this runner's case.

My mission in writing this book was to share my experiences with other runners so they could use what I've learned to train smarter, avoid injuries, and become the best runners they can be. Never give up, never stop trying, and never stop learning.

219. Know When It's Okay to Quit

Quit? Doesn't that fly in the face of what I just said? Not really.

Knowing when to quit is so important that it was hard to find the perfect place for it in this book. At first, this tip was in the competition chapter, but it's about far more than competition. Next, it was in the beginners' chapter, but even veterans need to be reminded that sometimes quitting is the smartest decision.

Then it occurred to me that this chapter would be the perfect place since juxtaposing it after a seemingly contradictory tip would jar readers into paying more attention to this advice.

In the culture of running, quitting has such a negative connotation that some runners and coaches probably had a knee-jerk reaction just reading the heading. Runners associate quitting with failure, but there are times when quitting is the right move.

In business, the most successful leaders know how to be flexible. When circumstances change, they can quickly change directions. In short, they know the importance of quitting when their actions aren't leading to the desired results.

How does this apply to runners? Because the mantra of running is "Don't quit," some runners are very inflexible when it comes to training. They attempt to struggle through a training run after an injury, making the injury worse. They're stubbornly inflexible about staying on schedule, even when they're sick or injured. Thousands of runners do marathons in hot weather, even when it carries a risk of permanent injury. They stick with training plans that don't work for them.

Sometimes, the smart business decision is to quit one approach and move to another. It's the same with running.

220. Never Stop Learning

When you're learning, you're growing. You may not be as fast as you once were, but you can still be smarter than you've ever been. Some of my friends are amazed by how much I know about running. I'm amazed by how little I know. Seldom does a day go by that I don't learn something new about my favorite sport.

Many years ago, I noticed that some people reached a point in their lives where they seemed to tire of learning. "This is the way the world is," they seemed to lament, "There's nothing I can do about it." You've seen these people. Seniors who seem to be locked into the 1950s, baby boomers who seem to be forever in the hippie 1970s, and Gen Xers who think that music died in the 1990s. Don' be like these people.

This is the single most important tip I'd like to leave with you. The world is a thrilling place. There is so much more to learn—even about a sport as simple as running. Never stop learning!

221. Live in the Moment

Hopefully, this book has entertained you and revealed some running wisdom you can use for the rest of your life. If you learned how to prevent just one major injury, you're a better runner than you were before reading it. And yet, in spite of over 200 pages of wisdom on running, we still haven't addressed a key question.

Why do we run?

Each runner would probably answer this question a different way. Some of us run for the competition to be the best we can be. Others run to lose weight. Millions run for the simplest of reasons—it's fun. So why do you run? One of my training partners put it this way.

I can't speak for anyone else, but at a certain point the joy of running surpassed by a pretty wide margin my desire to make sense out of it. I don't know why I run. I don't know why I race. I don't know why I compete. I don't need to know. Because running means more to me than curiosity. It goes deeper than knowledge. I run. I compete. I move on down the line. I'm a runner.

- Jeff Edmonds, 1st overall, Avenue of the Giants Marathon, 2009

It's easy to get carried away with training, pressures at work, or the need to lead the pack in that big workout. Pause for a moment and give thanks that you're able to run. You're fitter and healthier than coworkers who are 20 years younger. Look around you and see what everyone else is missing.

My dream is that this book will help you make running a lifelong passion, as it is for me. You are a runner. Live in the moment.

Run.

Recommended Readings

The Complete Guide to Running: How to be a Champion from 9 to 90 by Earl Fee

> If I could only recommend one book on running, it would be this one. It is quite simply the best book on training ever written for masters in the 400m, 800m, and 1500m, but it covers other distances as well. Every runner should have this book.

Daniels' Running Formula, 3rd Edition by Jack Daniels, PhD

> If you want to build your own training schedule or know the exact paces to run for intervals, tempos, and marathon workouts, this is the book for you. You will find training schedules for distances from the 5K to the marathon. If you're serious about racing, buy this book.

Training for Young Distance Runners by Larry Greene and Russ Pate

> Although this book is written from a coach's point of view, it contains a wealth of information that's extremely valuable to high school and middle school runners. Obviously, it's also a great resource for coaches.

About the Author

Grady Cash is a futurist and retired Certified Financial Planner who speaks professionally on running, healthy aging, and the seven stages of retirement. Grady was an average runner in 1999 when he suffered a near career-ending injury that kept him from running for two years. Upon returning to running, he vowed to never take his favorite sport for granted again. He immersed himself in every book he could find on running and trained under a 3-time Olympian. As a result, he propelled himself from average to one of the fastest runners in the world in his age group.

Grady has been world ranked in the 200, 400, and 800 meters. He holds the world record in the 4x400 meter relay in his age group. He has been the Tennessee Senior Games age group champion in every distance from 50 meters to 10,000 meters and has raced all distances from 50 meters to the ultramarathon. He has run the original marathon in Athens, Greece three times. He is a cyclist, weightlifter, and a tireless advocate and role model for healthy aging. He lives in Nashville, Tennessee. Meeting planners who wish to contact Grady for speaking engagements may do so through Facebook or at GradyCash@gmail.com.

NOTES

Printed in Great Britain
by Amazon

33183365R00136